DATE DUE

INSTRUMENTATION IN
SPEECH-LANGUAGE PATHOLOGY

Instrumentation in Speech -Language Pathology

Edited by Chris Code and Martin Ball

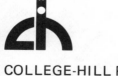

COLLEGE-HILL PRESS, INC.,
San Diego, CA 92105

© 1984 Chris Code and Martin Ball

College-Hill Press, Inc.,
4284 41st Street,
San Diego, CA 92105

Library of Congress Cataloging in Publication Data
Main entry under title:

Instrumentation in speech-language pathology.

   Bibliography: p.
   Includes index.
   1. Speech,Disorders of—Diagnosis. 2. Language
disorders—Diagnosis. 3. English language—Phonetics—
Instruments. I. Code, Christopher. II. Ball, Martin.
[DNLM: 1. Speech therapy—Instrumentation. 2. Phonetics.
WM 475 158]
RC423.I47   1984   616.85'5   83-26363
ISBN 0-933014-25-2

Note: This book is published outside the Americas and
US dependencies by Croom Helm Ltd, Provident House,
Burrell Row, Beckenham, Kent BR3 1AT, under the
title of *Experimental Clinical Phonetics: Investigatory
Techniques in Speech Pathology and Therapeutics*.

Printed and bound in Great Britain

CONTENTS

LIST OF CONTRIBUTORS

Evelyn Abberton, PhD, Lecturer in Phonetics, Department of Phonetics and Linguistics, University College, Gower St., London WC1E 6BT England.

James Anthony, PhD, Senior Lecturer in Phonetics, Department of Linguistics, University of Edinburgh, 40 George Square, Edinburgh EH8 9LL, Cleft Palate Unit, Royal Hospital for Sick Children, Edinburgh, Scotland.

Martin J. Ball, MA, Senior Lecturer in Linguistics and Phonetics, School of Speech Therapy, South Glamorgan Institute of Higher Education, Llandaff Centre, Western Avenue, Cardiff CF5 2YB Wales.

Daniel S. Beasley, PhD, Professor and Chairman, Department of Audiology and Speech Pathology, Memphis State University, Memphis, Tennessee 38105, USA.

Chris Code, PhD, Lecturer in Speech Pathology and Neurolinguistics, School of Speech Pathology, Leicester Polytechnic, Scraptoft Campus, Scraptoft, Leicester LE7 9SU England.

Steven E. Deutsch, PhD, Speech Pathologist, Audiology and Speech Pathology Service, Veterans Administration Medical Center, 5901, East Seventh St, Long Beach, California 90822, USA.

Alvirda Farmer, PhD, Associate Professor, School of Education, San Jose State University, San Jose, California 95192, USA.

Adrian J. Fourcin, PhD, Professor of Phonetics, Department of Phonetics and Linguistics, University College, Gower Street, London WC1E 6BT England.

Nigel Hewlett, PhD, Lecturer in Linguistics, Department of Speech Therapy, Queen Margaret College, Clerwood Terrace, Edinburgh EH12 8TS Scotland.

Walter H. Moore, PhD, Associate Professor, Communicative Disorders Department, California State University, Long Beach, California 90840, USA.

Daniel J. Orchik, PhD, Chief of Audiology, Shea Clinic, 1080 Madison Avenue, Memphis, Tennessee 38104, USA.

Linda L. Riensche, PhD, Assistant Professor, Department of Communication Disorders, University of New Mexico, Albuquerque, New Mexico 87134, USA.

Marcel A.A. Tatham, PhD, Professor of Linguistics, Cognitive Studies Centre, University of Essex, Wivenhoe Park, Colchester CO4 3SQ Essex, England.

PREFACE

Running parallel with developments in technique and methodology in experimental phonetics, have been advances in the investigation of speech production and perception in communication disorders. This has resulted in a mutually beneficial cross-fertilisation: pathology has benefited from the clinical application of the investigatory techniques of experimental phonetics, and our understanding of the mechanisms and processes of normal speech production and perception has been improved through research with various clinical populations. It is our intention to present in this volume contents that will serve as an up-to-date review, a source book, a laboratory handbook and a comprehensive introduction to current methods in experimental phonetics and their application in speech pathology and therapeutics. Accordingly, we have called this field *experimental clinical phonetics.*

We have aimed to bring together in one volume a collection of chapters, each devoted to one experimental or instrumental technique, which both introduces and surveys the application of that technique with the communicatively impaired. Each chapter describes a technique in non-technical terms, outlines its role in experimental phonetics and details its application and impact in speech pathology and therapeutics. As such the book should be of value to clinicians, researchers, lecturers and students in speech pathology, phonetics, linguistics and experimental psychology. It was also our intention to enlist contributors who were not simply eminent experimental phoneticians, but had direct experience, through research, teaching or clinical work, with the communicatively impaired.

The book presents a comprehensive coverage of major techniques. However, in planning such a book, it was inevitable that some techniques would be left out. The criteria for inclusion were that the technique had played a major role in experimental phonetics, had had widespread application in speech pathology, had a contribution to make to patient management and clinical decision making, was non-invasive and had contributed substantially to our understanding of communication disorders.

Speech is arguably the most interesting, and certainly one of the most complex and highly skilled behaviours that human beings are capable of, and breakdown in the production or perception of speech is not only a devastating handicap, but also of immense theoretical interest. It is our hope that this book will make both a practical and theoretical contribution to knowledge of communication disorders, and lead to wider utilisation of instrumental techniques by clinicians, to the benefit of both practitioner and patient.

C.C.
M.J.B.

1 RECORDING AND DISPLAYING SPEECH

Marcel A.A. Tatham

Introduction

The object of this chapter is to describe some of the methods available to us for recording and displaying speech signals. A quick glance at the titles of chapters in this book shows that speech signals are not simply the sounds of speech as picked up by a microphone. The investigation of speech, whether normal or pathological, involves examining many aspects of speaking other than the soundwave. In almost every case the particular aspect of speaking being investigated, whether the neuro-motor system, the aerodynamic system, the vocal-tract anatomy or configuration, or the acoustics of speech involves an instrumental technique which converts or transduces information or data about speech behaviour into electrical signals. Since any scientific investigation requires careful control and interpretation of the data there can be no question that it becomes very important to have some kind of permanent record of the phenomena under investigation, if only to repeat the experiment or check the validity of any inferences we might make. In work in speech we generally make two kinds of permanent record: (1) a recording of the actual data, obtained as closely as possible to the original conversion of the information into electrical signals, and (2) a visual recording of the final output of any electrical or other processing of the data for inspection and measuring by the investigator him or herself.

These days the first of these two permanent records is generally made on tape, and we shall see that there are various types of tape-recorder available to us for this purpose. The second of the permanent records is generally made as a tracing on strip chart paper, though there are other possibilities. The choices available to us must not be made randomly, however, or on some basis such as cost, since the wrong choice could easily result in distorted or destroyed data, or even incorrect results for the investigation. Choice among methods of recording and displaying speech signals has to be based on two major considerations: (1) the characteristics of the signal to be recorded or displayed, and (2) whether or not the characteristics of the recording

1

and displaying equipment match the signal's own characteristics. Clearly to make such a choice and to make the fullest use of the available equipment any researcher must have sufficient knowledge of the data and the equipment to avoid the random or incorrect use of equipment.

Recording Speech Data Signals

Tape-recorders

The first choice of a medium for recording data signals must be tape. Other media are available, such as disc and film which have been outdated, or solid-state recording (see below) which is not quite ready for widespread use in work in speech. The data holding medium is therefore the tape in a tape-recording system and this tape forms part of a mechanical system at the heart of the machine. It is important for the understanding of various types of tape-recorder to realise that basically a tape-recorder consists of three parts: (a) the recording electronics, (b) the mechanical system including the tape itself, and (c) the replay electronics.

Direct Recording. As far as we are concerned in speech research the limiting factor in the characteristics of tape-recording rests with the mechanical/tape system rather than with the electronics. The characteristics of the latter are generally sufficiently sophisticated to accommodate any speech signal. The actual process of getting the signal onto the tape, and keeping it there for replaying is however subject to some quite severe limitations which will have an effect on our instrumental methods.

1. The first parameter of tape-recorders I want to consider is that of signal-to-noise ratio. This is a way of expressing the difference between the amplitudes of the highest and lowest recordable signals. Since the dynamic range of speech signals of whatever kind rarely exceeds 50 dB, we might specify that our minimum requirement is for a signal-to-noise ratio of 50 dB (the decibel is a unit of amplitude). That is, if our highest amplitude signal is recorded just below some level which would introduce an unacceptable amount of distortion into the signal (thereby influencing any subsequent investigation of that signal) then the noise 'floor' inherent in any tape-recording should be at least 50 dB below that highest level.

2. The second important parameter of a tape-recording system is its frequency response. This refers to the machine's ability to record

and replay a particular frequency range without distorting the amplitude relationships within that range. Thus three tones, say, one at 400 Hz, another at 1 kHz and a third at 8 kHz of equal amplitude before recording must be reproduced after recording with their equal amplitudes preserved. This is why frequency response specifications must be stated with reference to ability to maintain this amplitude relationship. Generally a typical specification might be: 45 Hz to 18 kHz plus or minus 2 dB, meaning that over the frequency range stated amplitude relationships will be held on replay within a band 2 dB greater or 2 dB less than the amplitude of a reference tone at 1 kHz. Modern tape-recorders easily achieve this level of amplitude integrity provided they are kept well maintained.

However, it is important to note also that the ability of a tape-recorder to maintain amplitude integrity depends very much on the overall amplitude of the signal being recorded. A cassette tape-recorder using a good tape formulation would maintain the amplitude relationship in our example within 2 dB of the reference amplitude probably only if that reference amplitude were 20 dB lower than the maximum the machine could record at 1 kHz without more than the minimum of distortion. But raise the reference to that minimum distortion level (or 0 dB) and the same machine/tape combination might show a frequency response within 2 dB only over a range of 45 Hz to 8 or 9 kHz — insufficient for recording, say, the audio waveform of speech for the purpose of subsequent instrumental investigation. An open-reel tape-recorder on the other hand would have no difficulty holding amplitude integrity to its maximum recording level for this given frequency range.

This illustrates a major difference between open-reel and cassette tape-recorders. Their published frequency response specifications may often look identical, but usually for the cassette machine the reference level is 20 dB below the maximum level at which we will probably want to record. This means that high frequencies will play back with artificially reduced amplitude, making nonsense of any attempt to relate amplitude and frequency in a recording of the original signal; or it means that you have to keep down the level of the recording, greatly reducing the usable signal-to-noise ratio of the recorder — probably to a figure too narrow for our purposes. With the cassette recorder, because of its miniature dimensions, the position quickly worsens as the machine ages or if it is not scrupulously maintained in a good and clean condition, so that although it is true to say that high-frequency components of speech are generally low in amplitude anyway an element of doubt is introduced when using a tape-recorder that can only achieve the required frequency response at low amplitude settings.

Even with open-reel machines there is a general rule: better signal-to-noise ratios and better frequency response will be achieved with the widest tapes moving at the highest speeds. Consider that on a normal two-channel cassette recorder the width of each track is one quarter (two tracks in each direction) of one eighth of an inch (the tape width) moving at 1.875 in/s compared with a normal two-channel open-reel machine where the tracks are one half (two tracks in one direction only) of one quarter of an inch (the tape width) moving at 7.5 in/s (usually), or better at 15 in/s. It is the area of tape that passes across the recording and replay heads in a given time which is critical: the more the better. Less than one thirty-second of the area of tape passes under a recording head per track on a cassette machine in a given time than on an open-reel machine running at 15 in/s. There are a few cassette recorders available which run at a speed of 3.75 in/s which might just make acceptable recordings for instrumental analysis, but these are rare and problems of compatibility with other recorders arise.

3. Distortion in tape-recording is another parameter we must watch out for. In general the most disturbing form of distortion occurs when the oxide on the tape becomes magnetically saturated. This happens if we attempt to record a signal of too great an amplitude (see below). Most tape-recorders these days are satisfactory from this point of view provided no attempt is made to record a signal above the 0 dB reference point indicated on the machine's recording meters. Such a level should give a distortion level of less than 1 per cent which should not bother us unduly in subsequent analysis of the replayed signal.

FM Recording. The above description of the characteristics of tape-recorders refers to ordinary or direct-recording machines. The usual lowest frequency which can normally be recorded accurately is seldom below about 35 Hz. Many of the signals which we need to record for instrumental analysis however contain components below this frequency, and indeed may contain frequencies as low as 0 Hz; that is, may contain periods where there is no change in signal. Such steady-state signals are rather like the signal you would get by connecting two wires to a battery: a constant (not changing) amplitude around 1.5 volts. Speech signals which come into this category include the aerodynamic signals of air-pressure and airflow (see Chapter 5), glottograph signals (Chapter 4), some components of electromyography signals (Chapter 3), etc.

Under these conditions clearly an ordinary tape-recorder is going to be unsuitable for recording: it will simply fail to record low frequency signals or hopelessly distort them. Instead we usually use a machine which is different in as much as its electronics are preceded by circuitry designed to process or encode the incoming signal to make it suitable for normal recording.

The encoding process is known as frequency modulation (FM). The extra circuitry generates internally its own signal (called a carrier) which is well within the recording range of a normal tape-recorder. This new signal is then modulated or transformed using the incoming difficult signal. The result is that the original signal is modulated onto the internally generated signal in such a way that both can be recorded in the normal way. On playback, additional circuitry after the normal playback electronics decodes the speech signal back from the composite, modulated signal, rejecting the internally generated carrier, to output to an analysis or display device a copy of the original signal. Normally such FM tape-recorders accept and play back signals over the range 0 Hz to around 10 kHz, though wider frequency responses are often possible. Clearly it is important to know the frequency characteristics of the signal you wish to preserve on tape: if there are to be any signals with frequency components below the frequency response of a normal direct record tape-recorder then a FM machine must be used. Digital tape-recorders (see below) are also available which can record steady-state and low-frequency signals.

Noise Reduction. Many tape-recorders, especially cassette machines, incorporate (or make provision for the external connection of) a noise-reduction system, the most popular of which are Dolby B, C, HX and Professional HX, or dbx. All of these alter amplitude relationships in the incoming signal in order to compress a signal's dynamic range to allow the tape better to accommodate it. They are primarily designed for music recording where the dynamic range of the signal may well exceed 90 dB (much wider than the dynamic range of speech). On replay the compression is reversed to expand the recorded signal back to its original dynamic range. Provided the expansion is a perfect mirror image of the compression then in theory what comes out of the machine will be identical to what went in. In practice such an ideal situation is never achieved, and, depending on which noise reduction system is being used, amplitude/frequency integrity is more or less disturbed and several intrusive forms of distortion are introduced. For instrumental analysis of any speech signal (as opposed to just listening to a recording) the only advice possible is: do not use any noise reduction system. If your tape-recorder cannot achieve a better signal-to-noise ratio than, say, 50 dB (and many cassette machines, especially the portable ones, cannot) without the help of noise-reduction then the machine is simply unsuitable for any of the research techniques described in this book.

Digital Recording. All signals connected with speech (with the possible exception of some components of neurally-originating signals) are analog in form. That is, amplitude variations in the signals exhibit transitions which are smooth and continuous in nature. Digital tape-recorders, by contrast, expect to record signals by sampling the signal's amplitude level at particular discrete moments in time. For each time interval (or window) a number is recorded which is equivalent to a measurement of the average amplitude during the time interval sampled. The analog signal's smooth amplitude changes in time are therefore converted into discrete amplitude measurements which do not show that same smoothness, but which rather exhibit discontinuities of amplitude. This process of changing from smooth to discontinuous representation of amplitude is called analog-to-digital conversion.

Clearly the more often the machine looks at the incoming signal the less obtrusive will be any discontinuities. In general to capture a given frequency range a digital device needs to sample the input signal at a rate somewhat more than twice as often as the highest frequency in the incoming analog signal. So, if we expect speech to have its highest frequency component around 12 kHz, then it must be sampled at least 25,000 times per second. Fortunately no digital tape-recorder's analog-to-digital converter samples this slowly. They all accommodate input frequencies up to 20 kHz because all are basically designed to cover the entire range of human hearing (20 Hz to 120 kHz) and music signals. So, at least with digital tape-recorders we need not worry about frequency response. Similarly the dynamic range (expressed as bits) need not worry us; digital tape-recorders generally handle 14 bits (equivalent to a dynamic range of around 85 dB) or 16 bits (equivalent to a dynamic range of around 95 dB).

There are several standards current in digital tape-recorders. These are now settling down to three, differing standards being used for professional and domestic purposes. None of this need worry us from the point of view of a digital recorder's ability to record and reproduce signals for our purposes. But it does become important if tapes are to be interchanged between machines. The United States and Japan currently employ a slightly different (but totally incompatible) standard from that used in Europe for the type of machine which makes recordings on standard videocassettes. Make sure the machine used matches the one you want to play back on with respect (a) to sampling rate, and (b) to amplitude range (expressed as bits).

Digital studio recorders (usually open-reel) are somewhat different from domestic machines, and since the latter have a quality which on almost all fronts exceeds that of the best analog studio recorders hitherto available we can assume that for speech research the domestic types will be used. There are basically two types of domestic digital recorder available. Before looking at how they differ it is worth noting that there is no difference between a digital and an analog machine as far as connecting microphones, loudspeakers, headphones or other ancilliary equipment is concerned — ordinary analog signals are presented to the machine and, except for copying between recorders or connecting to other digital equipment, ordinary analog signals come out.

Both types of domestic digital tape-recorder use tape housed in cassettes. In one type the signals are recorded on the tape by scanning the moving tape diagonally by means of a rotating recording head. How this works need not worry us here; the method used is exactly the same as that used on most domestic videocassette recorders. Indeed the actual recording part of the machine (that part used to write the signal on the tape) is identical for all intents and purposes to a video machine, only the electronics before and after are different. These extra electronics are the analog-to-digital converter which makes our incoming analog signals digital, and the digital-to-analog converter which makes the played back digital signals analog again for output. It is possible to obtain these converters in a separate box for adding to a standard videocassette recorder to convert it into an audio machine. The tape used for both video and audio recording on this type of machine is identical and housed in identical cassettes whether of the VHS, Beta or Philips V2000 type.

The other type of digital cassette recorder uses cassettes roughly the size of the audio compact cassettes we are used to. They have narrower tape than the video-type machines described above, and do not use the scanning method of recording the signal onto the tape. Instead the tape is recorded linearly in much the same way as an ordinary recording is made linearly (except, of course, that we are recording numbers with digital machines). Here however the similarity ends, for a large number of tracks are recorded on the tape, each coping with a portion of the digital signal. Additional tracks are recorded for checking that errors in recording the digits are not occurring (or correcting them if they do occur); error checking and correction are always automatic, and so need not worry the user.

From the point of view of actual operation the digital machine should not be treated any differently from its analog counterpart, with the single exception that when recording it is extremely important not to try to record a signal of too high an amplitude: overload distortion on a digital tape-recorder is far, far worse than on an analog machine. Since however, the dynamic range of digital machines exceeds that of analog machines the recording controls can be kept down to make sure this does not happen.

As mentioned earlier, you will have no worries about the specifications of any digital tape-recorder you might encounter. All are much more than adequate for our purposes. One thing it is necessary to be aware of, though, is that editing (see below) on digital machines is quite different from editing on analog machines. Physical editing in the form of tape splicing is generally not possible at all, and electronic editing, whilst possible and extremely accurate, is difficult and requires expensive special equipment.

As digital machines become more common and it becomes appreciated that for a given price they are already, for a given quality, cheaper than their analog counterparts, it will be sensible to choose digital if both are available. Remember, though, that there are some problems of incompatibility which may be worth repeating. As far as domestic and semi-professional systems go there are two basic types which are not interchangeable: narrow tape linear recording and wide tape scanning recording. Particularly in the latter, sampling rates may vary between machines intended for use in Europe and those for use in the United States and Japan (the reason being that the sampling rate is tied to the video standards that the scanning system is based on and these video standards vary between Europe and the US/Japan). So, once again, play back on the same machine the recording is made on or at least on a machine built to the same standards. If material is to be sent to another person abroad, make sure the machine, if tied to video standards, is either basically compatible, or is a multi-standard machine.

Solid-state Recording

We looked above at the process of analog-to-digital conversion which constitutes the first stage in a normal digital tape-recorder. The tape is the medium for storage of the signals (in this case digital ones), but it should be clear that tape is not the only method by which signals can be stored. We are also familiar with the storage of analog signals on discs and optically on film, and there are also media in addition to tape for the storage of digital signals. In fact, though it may take another decade or so to be used for domestic music recording, there is a much better way of recording digital signals which does not rely on any mechanical or electro-magnetic method (such as disc or tape, respectively). This is known as solid-state recording.

Remember that the incoming analog signal to the tape-recorder was sliced by the analog-to-digital converter into time slots or samples, and that for each sample a measurement of amplitude was taken to provide a number; it was this number which was recorded. Solid-state recording simply places that number as one of a series of numbers associated with the string of samples into a computer-like memory involving no moving parts. At present such memories are limited by size and cost to perhaps the storage of one million samples. If we were sampling at, say, a rate of 25,000 times each second then one million memory samples would be sufficient for forty seconds' worth of recording. It is worth noting that the recording of music sampled at a rate of 40,000 times each second would require 84 million memory slots to record the average-length 35-minute symphony, or 432 million samples for a 3-hour opera!

Short samples of speech signals lasting just a few seconds, however, can easily be accommodated in available solid-state memories, and indeed it is this kind of recording which is used to hold the image on the screen of a storage oscilloscope (see below). I have been using a solid-state memory capable of holding just 256 samples for several years now, and found it invaluable.

Perhaps the most important advantage of such memories is that the sequence of numbers can be read out at any desired rate, once recorded. In the case of tape or disc storage of signals the readout is controlled mechanically (as is the recording) by the speed at which the medium (tape or disc) passes by the readout device (playback head in a tape-recorder, photo-sensor detecting reflected light from a laser in the case of a typical digital disc (Philips-Sony system)). In the case of solid-state recording readout rate is controlled by the rate at which each memory location is sequentially accessed for readout. Normally one would access the memory locations at the same speed as the original recording was made, but they can be accessed faster or slower for special purposes. One such purpose is the overcoming of high-frequency limitations in display devices such as chart recorders, where by accessing at half normal rates in effect the high-frequency response of the chart-recorder is doubled (see below).

A solid-state recorder is a special-purpose computer memory system. It is possible to use for the same purpose the memory of a general purpose computer, provided steps are taken to convert the usual analog signal into a digital version prior to feeding it into the computer. Placing the recording into the computer's own solid-state memory is no more difficult than using a purpose-built solid-state recorder, except that the computer must be programmed for the purpose. While we wait for large-scale memories in the recorders there is one advantage to using a computer. Provided the incoming signal is broken up time-wise into chunks of, say, one second's duration spaced by a blank period of, say, a further second, then the computer will have time during the blank period to dump or readout the contents of its memory (the previous 'active' period of signal) onto a further storage medium like, for example, a floppy-disk capable of holding much larger amounts of signal. This method of storing digital signals is used in a speech laboratory during experiments which involve a subject delivering brief responses to stimuli. While the subject is listening to the next stimulus the recording of his previous response is dumped onto the disk, clearing the memory for his next response. What is on the disk constitutes the recording.

A floppy-disk is either 5.25 or 8 inches in diameter and made of flexible plastic housed in a more rigid cardboard jacket. One or both surfaces of the disc are covered with magnetic oxide, and it is on this that the numerical information is recorded. Typically a 5.25 inch disk can hold 250,000 samples. Playback is in chunks back into the computer's memory, and then out via a digital-to-analog converter.

The Audio Recording Session

Making the Recording

The majority of recordings the speech pathologist will make in the course of his/her duties or research will be of the audio waveform of patients and of normal speech for comparison purposes. There are good ways and bad ways of making a recording, especially when the material is to be analysed instrumentally. Listening to a recording will not normally provide a very good judgment as to its quality. The reason for this is quite simple: a subjective impression will tend to overlook the imperfections in any recording, unless they are very gross, but these imperfections will show up all too readily in any instrumental analysis that might follow. This may lead to difficulties and inaccuracies in measurements. The only way to ensure a good recording is to know what factors influence the quality of recordings, and try to make sure you have obtained the most satisfactory conditions possible.

Location. Echo is one of the biggest problems likely to be encountered. Ideally recording should be made in a studio especially designed for audio. Unfortunately this is going to be available to very few clinicians. The next best thing is to select the quietest, most heavily furnished room possible, and preferably one certainly no larger than the average-sized living room. The idea is that heavy furnishings (particularly soft chairs, carpets and drapes) serve to absorb unwanted reflections that bare walls, floor, windows and ceiling would normally produce, and in addition to provide some kind of insulation against noises coming into the room from outside. Listen carefully for such unwanted noises. Normally we tend not to notice them ourselves, but the microphone will mercilessly pick them up. Listen out especially for the noise of people walking along corridors, aircraft and traffic noise, and particularly for the drone of air-conditioning systems. These have become so much a part of our lives that it is common to be surprised on hearing a recording of 'silence' made in a room prone to these noises.

Microphones. Having chosen the quietest, least reverberant (or deadest) room you can find, further obtruding echoes and outside noises can be minimised by carefully selecting microphones and using them properly. Omnidirectional microphones (which pick up sound from all around them) are usually not suitable — after all the signal is usually coming from just one direction: from the lips of the subject. Choose a directional microphone and make sure it is pointing roughly at the subject (though not in such a way that he blows onto it directly, but talks across it). There is no need to go into the vast array of types of microphone available; most these days, except the very cheapest, are good enough and there is little point in spending hundreds.

Select a microphone which has a reasonably flat frequency response over the speech range (say, 75 Hz to 12 kHz plus or minus 3 dB). There is one kind of reliable and excellent microphone which satisfies almost all the conditions we could impose for recordings of the kind we intend to make. This is the battery-powered electret microphone mounted with a lapel clip or slung on a cord round the neck. Choose the directional type. Such a microphone has the additional advantage that almost automatically you are likely to mount it in precisely the right place — around 15 inches from the subject's mouth, not immediately in front of him (to avoid breath noises), and not on some reverberant surface like a table. In fact the only disadvantage with this kind of microphone is the possible pickup of the rustle of clothes, but this should not be too difficult to take care of.

One further point on microphones: it is often necessary to record a conversation between two or more people, say between the clinician and patient. In this case you must use two microphones connected preferably to the two separate channels of a stereo recorder. In this way you will find that on playback it is very easy to keep the two signals almost entirely separate with just enough 'breakthrough' for you to hear what is going on by listening to just one channel if necessary. If more than two people are to be recorded, then the best practice is to have a microphone for each, with the signals mixed electronically using a microphone mixer before recording on one or two channels. I do not recommend placing a single omnidirectional microphone on a table in the middle of a group of subjects: almost every rule of recording technique is violated by the practice, as you will find out when you come to analyse such a recording!

Stereo recorders are readily available these days to provide two-track recording as described above. If, however, you are going to do a lot of group recording you should seriously consider one of the semi-professional four-track machines. Anything more than four tracks, though possible (32- and 64-track recorders do exist) becomes prohibitively expensive.

One word of warning. Compatibility between recorders is not guaranteed, and you should be careful to ensure you can play back recordings either on the machine used for making them or on another machine you have previously tested for compatibility. Do not rely on specification sheets to indicate compatibility — two identical tape-recorders (particularly of the cassette type) can have slightly different alignment of the record and playback heads which will make tapes recorded on the one reproduce badly on the other.

Using the Gain Control. Avoid at all costs automatic gain controls for recording. These come labelled in several different ways, so if in doubt consult a competent engineer to ask whether (a) automatic gain control (often called AGC) is used on the machine, and (b) how to switch it out. The trouble with automatic gain control is that although such a system takes much of the work out of making a recording it will considerably distort the amplitude relationships of the recordings you make, to say nothing of attempting faithfully to record the background noise you have gone to such pains to remove.

Having decided never to use AGC, you are now faced with using the manual gain control for recording. Imagine that a tape-recorder looks at the amplitude of sound through a window. That window has a top and a bottom. This top and bottom are represented on the meter used in conjunction with the gain control. The window top is marked 0 dB and corresponds to the point where the meter scale usually changes to red (this applies both to meters like dials with pointers and the newer luminous displays). The bottom of the window is the far left of the meter (or bottom if it is mounted vertically). If you have the gain control too low the signal will be at the bottom of the window and insufficiently 'seen' by the recorder. On the other hand if you have the gain control too high then the signal will overshoot the window resulting in considerable unwanted distortion – again as unusable recording. The control must be manipulated to get the signal within the window.

How do you do this? Consider what speech sound is again for a moment. It has a certain amplitude range, and we already know that most tape-recorders can cope with that range. Some sounds have more amplitude than others, so logically the trick is going to be to set the gain control such that the loudest sounds just kick the needle to the 0 dB mark (or just light up that portion of the fluorescent display next to the 0 dB mark), and leave the rest to get on with itself. So how do we know what the loudest sound is going to be before it has happened? Research shows that the speech sound usually with the highest intrinsic amplitude is the [a] sound in a word like *cart*. If possible get the subject to say this sound, or a word containing this sound, several times into the microphone before you begin the recording session proper. Adjust the gain control carefully so that the meter just registers 0 dB, and no more. Make sure the subject is talking in what you expect to be a normal voice (practise him/her with using a microphone beforehand to make the voice as normal as possible).

And now most importantly: once you have set the gain control before the actual session begins do not touch it again, unless you can see during the session that you had obviously set it wrong. The point here is that the gain control improves or worsens the recorder's sensitivity to signals. If you change the setting during the recording, you will not be able to compare the amplitudes of anything recorded before the change with those of anything recorded after the change –

and you may want to do this. If it is absolutely necessary to make a change and the session cannot be restarted then do so deliberately and quickly, making a note of what you did and when you did it. Preferably start the session over again.

Listening to a Recording

No tape-recorder with a built-in loudspeaker is good enough for listening purposes, except for the crudest monitoring. To listen seriously to any recording you need the highest fidelity playback system available or affordable. Only the best systems will accurately preserve the amplitude and frequency relationships which make up the speech you are trying to listen to. Failing a good loudspeaker system use headphones. The fidelity of headphones can often be deceptive; they sound better than they really are objectively. But many people prefer them for auditory analysis purposes because, by putting you in more intimate touch with the signal being replayed, some find that concentration on listening is much better and that it is easier to be more objective in making judgments of what is being listened to. It's really up to you which you prefer, but try to ensure the best fidelity possible. Once again it's a question of looking for the flattest adequate frequency response curves.

Tape Editing

Editing of tape is often called for. This generally arises when portions of a recording need to be removed, or sections from several different recordings need to be put together onto a single tape. There are two ways of doing this: one is by physically cutting the tape and splicing together again in the required arrangement, and the other is to accomplish the same thing by electronic means. Cutting and splicing tape is a very time consuming business and can really only be done successfully if the original recording is made in the open-reel format at as high a tape speed as possible (to give the most room for locating the edit point on the tape). If you do go in for physically editing the tape in this way, make sure you get plenty of practice beforehand and never edit your original recording (you may make a mistake and destroy it). Always work on a copy of the tape. That way if you mess things up, you just make another copy and begin again. Remember though that copying tape results in degradation of the signal, so you must have an exceptionally clean recording to begin with. Furthermore if your final spliced tape contains many joins or is to be kept for more than a few weeks, you cannot guarantee that your splices will hold and a copy of the edited tape must be made. You will then work from this final copy. Note, though, that this final tape is a copy of a copy, with attendant multiplied degradation. (Incidentally, we can note here that degradation caused by copying does not happen with digital recordings unless there are multiple errors in the digits recorded.)

Electronic editing is to be preferred to physically splicing tape. This is done by connecting two tape-recorders together taking the signal out from the machine holding the original tape and into the second machine. Painstakingly the required portions of the original recording must be found by careful listening, and then copied onto the new tape on the second recorder with its controls set to record.

Displaying Speech Data Signals

The output of instruments used for analysis in the laboratory generally needs to be presented in some visual form. Sometimes all that is required is a temporary presentation for the purposes of monitoring during an experiment or, for example, for finding one's place in a recording prior to making some kind of permanent record of the data. For such temporary visual presentation purposes we usually use an oscilloscope, whereas for permanent visual recordings a strip chart-recorder is more usual.

Non-permanent Displays

Oscilloscopes. In general any oscilloscope (scope) will meet adequate standards for presentation of speech data provided that it has been maintained within its specification. Choices are between those scopes which show the data on a screen as it arrives and those which can be made to hold a portion of the data on the screen for more careful inspection. Storage scopes, as the latter are called, contain within them a solid-state memory which is constantly being fed with the incoming signal. At any one moment some previous portion of the data is held in the memory. Often the amount of data the memory can hold can be varied, but suppose the memory is set to hold one second's worth of data. On command (either from a switch on the front panel, or instruction from a computer) the scope will stop displaying the incoming signal and instead display the contents of its memory (the previous one second's worth) as a frozen image on the screen, until instructed to continue with the incoming data. A storage scope is an ordinary scope which contains a short solid-state memory. These memory devices are available separately for converting a non-storage scope into a storage one.

Generally the display portion of the scope consists of a cathode ray tube (CRT), but we are beginning to see now electronic displays of a quite different kind: liquid crystal displays (LCDs). These promise to be more accurate and to overcome some of the problems associated with CRT devices (one in particular being that CRTs are not very good for fast transients); such problems do not arise with the LCD.

Scopes able to display more than one trace at a time can be useful for comparing data on two (or sometimes more) separate channels, as can scopes able to display separate incoming signals in different colours, or varying intensities of a single signal in different colours.

Generally the screens of scopes are small in size (5 in diagonal measurement being perhaps the commonest). This does not make for convenience when a large number of people wish to view the screen at the same time. Large screen displays are possible, but it must be remembered that the larger the screen the worse the accuracy of the display. For serious measurement work from a scope display the large screens should be avoided.

In the case of CRT display scopes there are several alternatives available for the actual characteristics of the screen itself. The image is made on the screen by causing a phosphorescent material to glow by bombarding it in the right place with a beam of electrons. Variations are possible in the phosphor to produce (a) different colours of display, and (b) different characteristics of fading of the image (called persistence) once bombardment has stopped. These variations are possible by having different tubes fitted to the scope. The trick is to arrange for a phosphor which will not fade too quickly, but which will not fade so slowly as to cause blurring of the image. I myself use tubes which display the signal as a blue image which fades very quickly to leave a much fainter trace for a couple of seconds in yellow. The speed is there to avoid blurring (one simply concentrates on the blue colour), but continuity of display is maintained in the yellow afterglow. CRTs with these characteristics are available to fit most currently available CRT-type scopes. Although these variations are not yet available in the new LCD types we can expect to see these and other possibilities fairly soon.

The image on the screen of a scope vanishes almost immediately, or, if the storage type is in use, will vanish as soon as the memory is cleared. Permanent records of what has been on the screen can be obtained, either by photographing the screen, or, in the case of some storage scopes, arranging for the contents of the memory to be dumped onto some device capable of generating hard copy (permanent recording on paper of some kind). Photography, while useful in some instances, is not particularly to be recommended, although very high quality results are obtainable. For photography the camera is mounted usually at a fixed distance from the screen and hooded from its lens to the screen to prevent stray ambient light casting reflections on the screen itself. Film used in the camera is either a normal high-contrast type requiring developing and printing (so you do not know how successful your photography has been until these processes have been carried out), or of the instant-print kind (Polaroid or Kodak). The latter can be quite expensive if many prints are required of the display.

Permanent Displays

Sooner or later any recording of data, whether it be audio or some other kind of speech signal, will need to be inspected visually from a permanent record. Apart from the rather limited use of photography of the screen of a scope the most convenient method of providing a visual display which is permanent is to apply the signal to a chart recorder to give a permanent visual trace or record on paper. There are several kinds of chart recorder available, each, once again, with different characteristics which need careful examination so that the right one is chosen for the job in hand.

Pen Recorders. As with most chart recorders a pen recorder consists of an electronic section and a mechanical section. The electronics of the various types of recorder do not differ much, but the mechanical parts vary considerably and sometimes severely limit the machine's capabilities. Pen recorders have pens (usually of the felt-tipped variety) mounted in such a way that they impinge on paper which is made to unroll mechanically under the pen. There can be several pens, one for each channel of data to be recorded. The pen is made to move from side to side as the paper is unrolled, to inscribe a trace on the paper. The movement of the paper corresponds to the horizontal movement of the trace on the screen of a scope and the sideways movement of the pens corresponds to the vertical movement of the trace on the scope. Pen movement is wholly mechanical using electromagnets to cause sideways movement of the mounting of the pen. Two limiting factors are introduced: the weight of the mounting being moved, and the friction between the pen and paper. These combine to restrict the frequency response of the pen recorder to a range often no greater than 0 to 100 Hz. This is clearly insufficient for the vast majority of uses we would need for a chart recorder in the laboratory.

Ink-jet Recorders. One step up from the pen-recorder is the ink-jet recorder. These have been in common use in speech laboratories for around a quarter of a century. Instead of a pen marking the chart paper as it is mechanically unrolled a jet of ink is directed toward the paper literally spraying a trace. The nozzle of the jet is mounted in such a way that it can be deflected from side to side by electromagnets responding to the signal applied to the recorder (the signal we want to display). Because the mounting of the nozzle is lighter than that in a pen recorder and because there is no friction effect between jet and paper the frequency response of the recorder is greatly extended beyond what is possible with pen recorders. Normally we would expect a response from 0 to between 800 and 1000 Hz, and this is sufficient for most applications in the speech laboratory (though not of course for displaying all details of the audio waveform). An advantage of both pen recorders and ink-jet recorders is that the paper used is ordinary and cheap.

The effective frequency response of pen and ink-jet recorders can be extended by playing the signal to be displayed at half- or quarter-speed on the tape-recorder. Halving the speed of the tape-recorder effectively doubles the frequency response of the chart recorder, and so on. Note though that some distortion of lower frequencies is almost certain to occur using this method with an analog tape-recorder.

A new kind of ink-jet recorder is becoming available, though not quite yet in a form suitable for our work. In these machines ink is sprayed from a nozzle onto paper in the way described above, except that instead of oscillating the nozzle by using electromagnets, the jet of ink itself is oscillated by employing its own magnetic properties within a magnetic field set up around the jet in a way analogous to the deflecting of the electron beam in a CRT. This system is currently being used for drawing pictures and composing type on non-moving paper, but its possibilities for strip-chart recording are enormous. Since the mechanical inertia introduced by deflecting the nozzle in ordinary ink-jet recorders is removed the frequency range possible with these new machines is considerably widened to way beyond anything we would need as a maximum in the speech laboratory.

UV Recorders. Ultra-violet (UV) recorders use a very narrow beam of ultra-violet light to write the tracing representing the waveform of the incoming data signal on paper which is photo-sensitive in the ultra-violet region. A strong lamp generates the light and a system of mirrors and lenses focus it into one or more beams (depending on how many channels the recorder can display). Each beam is caused to fall on a tiny mirror mounted in such a way that electromagnets controlled by the incoming signal cause oscillations in the reflected beam. This oscillating beam is then made to fall on the unrolling photo-sensitive paper exposing it to leave an as yet undeveloped tracing. Exposing the paper to strong light develops the image.

Even with the very latest emulsions the traces on UV-sensitive paper are not entirely permanent and over a period of time will fade, especially if exposed to strong sunlight. Earlier images could be fixed by immersion in a bath of fixer and then washed and dried. An alternative method is to use an aerosol of fixer which is sprayed directly onto the paper and left to dry. These aerosols often also stain the paper yellow which improves the contrast of the image particularly for photo-copying purposes.

The main advantage of UV recorders is their wide frequency response, attainable easily as far as 15 kHz and beyond. Their main disadvantage is the quality of the image and the enormous cost of the photo-sensitive paper compared with the cheap ordinary paper used in pen and ink-jet recorders.

Fibre-optic Recorders. Also using photo-sensitive paper are the fibre-optic recorders. These collect light from a bright lamp housed within the recorder using a bundle of fibre optics. The tiny fibres are fanned out into a fine array mounted across and slightly above the photo-sensitive paper as it is mechanically unrolled. The appearance of light at the end of any one particular fibre optic is electrically controlled in sympathy with the amplitude variations in the incoming data signal. As with UV recorders a very wide frequency response is possible with these machines as well as the ability (not required in the speech laboratory for most purposes) to reproduce intermediary grey tones between black and white. Though unusual and perhaps over-specified for our purposes these machines are becoming more common and cheaper.

Thermal Recorders. Thermal recorders may have a promising future in the speech laboratory. They work by applying the incoming data signal to an array of very fine heat-generating elements placed in contact with the unrolling paper. The paper itself is heat sensitive and colour (usually blue or black) is revealed whenever the paper comes into contact with a heated element. As with fibre-optic recorders there are no moving parts (except for the unrolling paper) to limit frequency response of the system. With both types of recorder the actual limiting factor is the number of elements (either fibre-optics or heating elements) which can be packed into the array spread across the paper.

Conclusion

These are the main points I have been making in this chapter covering the means of recording and displaying speech signals:

1. Be sure you are fully aware of the characteristics of the speech signals you wish to record and display.

2. Choose the right machine for the recording job in hand, making sure in particular that you understand the limitations of cassette recorders.

3. If possible now, and certainly in the future, use a digital recorder. You will never have any worries about quality if you do, though editing may be difficult. Failing a digital recorder open-reel analog is to be preferred to standard cassette analog.

4. Check the frequency range of your data signal. If there are components lower than around 35 Hz you will need a frequency modulation tape-recorder or digital machine designed for the purpose.

5. For display purposes once again you must consider the characteristics of your data signal. Aerodynamic, audio amplitude, fundamental frequency, electromyography, etc. signals have narrow enough ranges (all within 0 to 1000 Hz) for adequate presentation on a cheap-to-run ink-jet recorder. Full details of the audio waveform (75 Hz to 12 kHz) can only be appreciated however on, for example, a UV recorder.

2 SPECTROGRAPHY

Alvirda Farmer

Introduction

Since its development in the late 1940s, the sound spectrograph or sonograph analyser has been the single most useful device for the quantitive analysis of speech. While early applications of the spectrograph were focused on the parameters of normal speaking patterns (Potter, Kopp and Kopp, 1966; Lehiste, 1967), this instrument has more recently been used to study just about every speech and language disorder.

Figure 2.1: A 6061 Sona-Graph Basic Spectrograph (a) and the recently introduced 7800 Digital Sona-Graph (b)

(a)   (b)

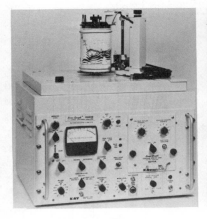 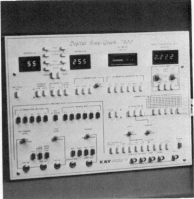

Source: Courtesy of Kay Elemetric.

The spectrograph (Figure 2.1a and 1b) performs a complex Fourier analysis of the speech signal, but the operation of the instrumentation

Figure 2.2: Narrow-band (a) with amplitude display and broad-band (b) with waveform spectrograms of 'aha'. Fo is estimated from the centre of the first /a/. For the narrow-band spectrogram the 5th harmonic is 8mm from the baseline and the 10th harmonic is 16mm from the baseline. Each computes (times 77 Hz/mm) to approximately 123 Hz.

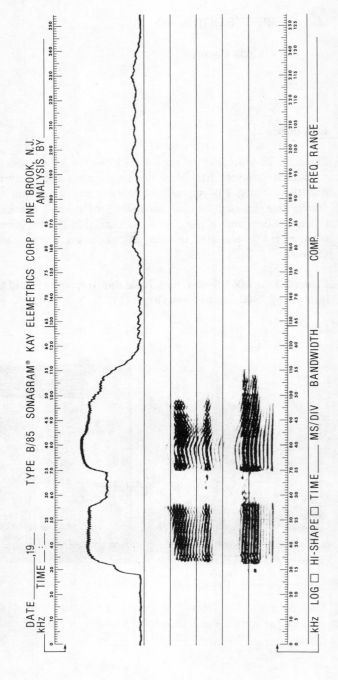

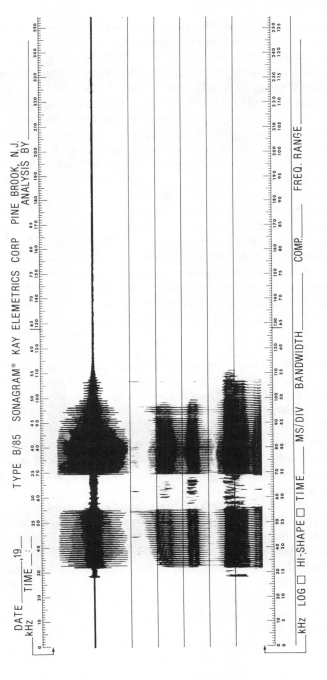

Source: Courtesy of Kay Elemetric.

is less complex and much safer than driving a car. Typically, a spectrograph includes a system to record acoustic signals on a loop or drum so that the recording may be rapidly and repeatedly replayed. A filter system scans the playback through successive (low to high) frequency bands. Sound energy in each frequency band is burnt onto a chemically treated paper by a stylus. Level of energy or intensity at each frequency is marked by darkness (high intensity) or lightness (low intensity). The completed spectrogram displays time on the abcissa (horizontal) and frequency on the ordinate (vertical). As shown in Figure 2.2, narrow (45 Hz) or broad (300 Hz) filters may be used for measuring frequency or duration and quality, respectively.

The ability to interpret the spectrogram will partially depend on understanding how it is produced. Further details describing the instrumentation and interpretation of spectrograms may be found in a variety of sources (Potter *et al.*, 1966; Lehiste, 1967; Agnello, 1975; Shoup and Pfeifer, 1976; Lieberman, 1977; Borden and Harris, 1980). This chapter will review clinical applications of the basic spectrograph. However, the development of new models and additional functions are available, and specific use of these are described in literature made available by the manufacturer.

Duration

One of the most frequent uses of the spectrograph is to examine speech segment durations. Visual cues for many sounds and sound contexts are often relatively unambiguous (for example, stop consonant-vowel-stop consonant). However, some segment boundaries are difficult to specify (glide-vowel-glide). Shoup and Pfeifer (1976) provide a list of major cues which may be used as boundary indicators between vowels and adjacent consonants. Since the visual contrast between segments varies, it is prudent carefully to design speech stimuli which measure the desired parameters and are clearly visible.

After Lisker and Abramson's (1964) classic study using voice onset time (VOT) to delineate voicing contrasts across languages, VOT has been used to study a variety of speech and language disorders. VOT is defined by Lisker and Abramson as the difference in time between the release of complete articulatory constriction and the onset of quasi-periodic vocal fold vibration. Examples of VOT modes are shown in Figure 2.3. Generally, VOT has been applied to stop consonants. However, the voicing contrasts of fricatives may also be compared (Code and Ball, 1982).

Vowel duration (VD) is another parameter which can be precisely

Figure 2.3: The VOTs are shown for /bu/ (left) and /pu/ (right). Amplitude display is also shown.

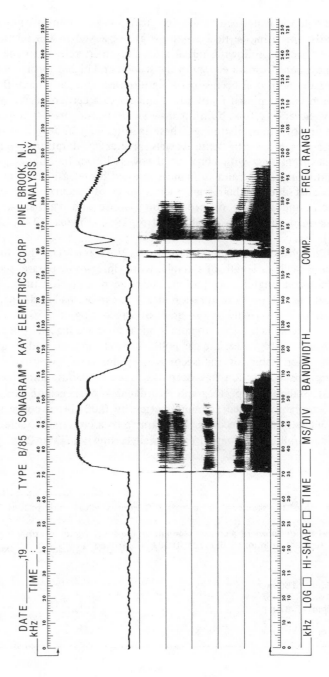

Source: Courtesy of Kay Elemetric.

measured. VD is defined as the distance from the point in time where regularly appearing vertical striations are observed in the second and higher formants following initial stop consonant release to the point in time where formant energy in the second and higher formants end in association with oral occlusion of the terminal stop consonant. Because duration is a temporal feature it is subject to a certain degree of variability. Several factors, both intrinsic and extrinsic, operate to produce variations of duration timing. These factors include, degree of vocalic laxness/tenseness with tense vowels greater in duration; degree of openness/tenseness with constricted vowels longer in duration; degree of diphthongisation; and influences exerted by releasing and arresting consonants due to their segmental features of voicing, place of production, and manner of production (House and Fairbanks, 1953; Zimmerman and Sapon, 1958; Delattre, 1962; Umeda, 1975; Lehiste, 1976).

Although not as frequently applied as VOT and VD, other duration measures such as length of syllable, word, interword, phrase, sentence and non-meaningful vocalisations have been used to study various populations. All of these duration measures can be made using a measuring rule of a wide-band spectrogram of a recording of a 50 Hz calibration tone. On such a spectrogram vertical lines are spaced 20 ms apart. For visual convenience, a clear millimetre rule can be used to prepare a conversion table of milliseconds to millimetres. Another way of making this conversion has been described by House and Fairbanks (1953). Since their spectrograph recorded 2.4s of speech on 318.5 mm, they simply multiplied the millimetres by 0.00754 to convert from millimetres into milliseconds. An example of a conversion table which provides a millimetre to millisecond scale is shown in Table 2.1.

Table 2.1:

The length of the spectrogram paper is 318.5mm which is equal to 2.4s in duration.

To find the *duration* of a chosen segment on the spectrogram multiply the length of the segment (in mm) by 0.00754 (0.00754 is arrived at by $\frac{318.5}{2.4} = 0.00754$).

Examples:

20mm	=	150 ms
10mm	=	75 ms
5mm	=	37 ms
3mm	=	22 ms
1mm	=	7 ms

Frequency

The spectrograph provides several frequency measures which have been used to study the acoustic signal of speech. These include fundamental frequency, formant frequency and antiresonance. While frequency information is visually less easy to measure than duration parameters, spectrograms include frequency calibration markings which simplify this process. Further clarification may be achieved by constructing a frequency calibration template on clear plastic which extends the markings across the spectrogram.

Fundamental frequency (Fo) is directly related to the vibration of the vocal folds and can be measured in two ways. If a male speaker has low enough Fo, then the individual vertical striations which correspond to glottal pulses may be visibly separated as shown in Figure 2.4. These striations can be counted between designated time periods and converted by the formula Fo equals the number of glottal pulses per timing marker divided by the time period between markers. If the speaker's Fo is too high for the vertical striations to be visibly separated for easy counting, then one may use a narrow-band spectrogram to determine Fo. In order to do this, one takes the value of the fifth or tenth harmonic and divides it by five or ten, respectively. Refer back to Figure 2.1 of the narrow-band spectrogram to estimate the Fo of the speaker using this method.

Formant Behaviour

The speaking voice is heard as the Fo and its harmonics which are multiples of the Fo. Some of the harmonics are emphasised because of the resonant characteristics of the vocal tract. These high energy harmonics are called formants. While most voices have several formants, clinical research has generally been concerned with F1 and F2. F1 is related more to manner of articulation in vowel consonant transitions and F2 is related more to place of articulation in vowel consonant transitions (Delattre, Liberman and Cooper, 1955). The frequencies of the formants may be predicted by three factors: the degree of constriction created by the height of the tongue; the distance from the larynx at which this constriction occurs; and the amount of lip-rounding, lip-protrusion or lip-spreading present (Stevens and House, 1955). Consequently, the relationship or distance between F1 and F2 has been used to describe the normal production of vowels (Peterson and Barney, 1952; Eguchi and Hirsh, 1969). Formant frequencies are identified by locating the approximate centre of the formant bars on wideband spectrograms and drawing a line through the formant at this point.

Figure 2.4: Spectrogram of 'cat' with Waveform. Fo is computed from the centre of the vowel by counting the vertical striations for 10ms. Since 7 vertical striations occurred in 10ms, Fo can be estimated at 70 Hz.

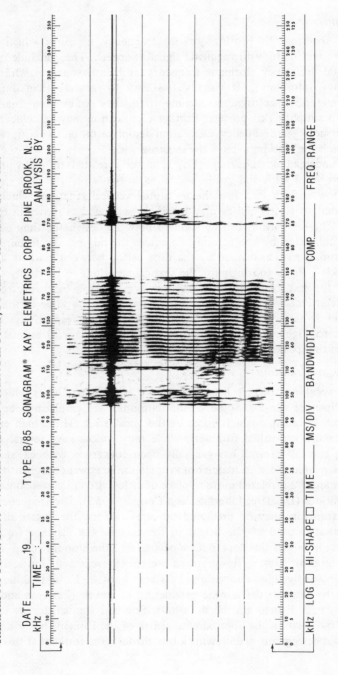

Source: Courtesy of Kay Elemetric.

Estimate of the centre measure of the formant is made using a conversion of Hz into millimetres. After the millimetre measure is made, reconversion into Hz completes the measure.

Antiresonance

Antiresonance may result from extra leakage of the vocal tract such as nasalisation which causes a major reduction in the magnitude of the envelope of the speech spectrum (Shoup and Pfeifer, 1976). Schwartz (1971) lists the four main features of vowel spectra in nasalised speech. They include: (1) reduction in intensity of the first formant; (2) presence of one or more antiresonances in the spectrum; (3) presence of extraresonances or presence of reinforced harmonics at frequencies at which energy is not normally expected; (4) a change or shift in the centre frequencies of formants.

Vocal Quality

Vocal abnormalities are visually apparent on the spectrogram and may include lack of vocalisation, extraneous vocalisation, intermittent vocalisation, sudden pitch breaks, loss of harmonic components and added noise components. Figure 2.5 provides examples of some vocal abnormalities. Since vocal abnormalities are visually obvious, discrete measures are generally not made from spectrograms. However, narrative descriptions of features are used to explain the acoustic patterns.

Applications in Speech Pathology

As mentioned earlier, almost every speech and language disorder has been studied via the spectrograph. This section will review a sample of the literature to demonstrate the uses of the spectrograph in speech pathology research. Disorders will be discussed by their generic medical model classifications as this approach may appeal to the clinician who is beginning to apply the spectrograph as a diagnostic instrument in evaluating a particular disorder.

Stuttering and Cluttering

By definition (Van Riper, 1971, p. 15) 'a stuttering behavior consists of a word improperly patterned in time and the stutterer's reaction thereto.' The spectrograph has permitted a careful analysis of speech segment duration for fluent and non-fluent speech in stutterers.

Agnello (1975) summarised several studies comparing VOT in

Figure 2.5: An Example of Vocal Abnormalities in Hoarseness (a). This speakers' production of 'ah' includes intermittent vocalisation, loss of harmonic components and antiresonance. A comparison (b) of hypernasal 'ah' (left) and normal 'ah' (right).

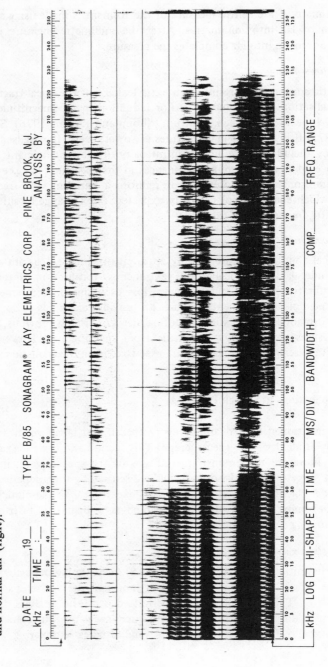

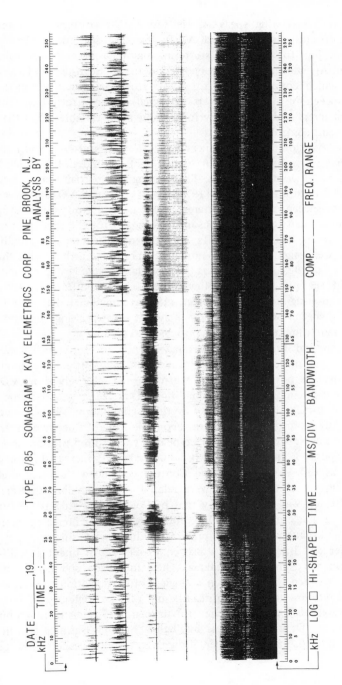

Source: Courtesy of Kay Elemetric.

normal and stuttering speakers. He found that stuttering children had significantly longer bilabial VOTs than non-stuttering children, which led him to suggest that stuttering may be a phonetic transition problem. Agnello's study was supported by that of Seebach and Caruso (1979) which compared VOT for all six stop consonants during the fluent speech of young stutterers with that of a control group. The eight stutterers had consistently longer and more variable VOTs than did the eight control subjects.

While Agnello found differences between adult stutterers and non-stutterers on voice termination time (VTT), he did not find VOT differences between the groups. This finding was partially confirmed by Metz, Conture and Caruso (1979a) who compared VOTs between the fluent speech of adult stutterers and a control group on six stop consonants and twelve stop consonant blends. With the exception of /tr/, stutterers had longer VOTs than did non-stutterers. Mean differences were significant for /b, br, bl, p, pr, tw/. Further, with the exception of /lg, kw/ stutterers showed larger standard deviations than did the non-stutterers. However, since mean differences were generally non-significant, Metz *et al*. (1979a) concluded that VOT in the fluent speech of adult stutterers may not serve as a single criterion for differentiating stutterers from normal speakers.

Brayton and Conture (1978) analysed VD in stutterers' speech under normal, noise and rhythmic stimulation conditions. They found that under the normal condition, stutterers had relatively short VDs and were disfluent. In the noise condition VD increased and disfluency decreased. Finally, when reading to rhythmic stimulation, VD increased significantly from that of the normal condition and disfluency decreased to its lowest level. They also compared vocal sound pressure level across conditions and found that it did not vary with increased fluency as well as did VD. Brayton and Conture concluded that temporal changes in speech production were related to fluency in stutterers. Their research was supported by that of Colcord and Adams (1979) who found that during singing VD, but not vocal SPL, increased significantly and that stutterers were predictably fluent while singing.

Farmer and Brayton (1979) also compared VD in fluent and disfluent Down's Syndrome speakers. They found no significant differences between the groups on a single word articulation test. However, the groups differed significantly on VD, intelligibility in conversational speech and frequency of disfluency. The disfluent group had shorter VDs and were less intelligible in conversational speech. They concluded that the disfluent Down's Syndrome speakers showing disfluency and poor intelligibility in connected speech were displaying cluttering behaviour. Farmer, Hambly and Jackson (in progress) are presently comparing VD between learning disabled children who clutter and controls.

Spectrography analysis has shown that speech segment timing differs in stuttering and cluttering. The relationship between long and variable VOTs and shorter than normal VDs in the stuttering population is interesting and should raise a number of questions for further research in both populations. Further, these findings indicate a method of objectively documenting speech parameter changes which may occur in the successful treatment of stuttering. It would appear that at post-treatment fluent stutterers should exhibit shorter VOTs and longer VDs than they had in their pre-treatment disfluent speech. One such study (Metz, Onufrak and Ogburn, 1979b) has shown that after a period of treatment, VDs and the occurrence of voicing during stop consonant production increased significantly in stutterers.

Dysarthrias

Perhaps the most frequent use of the spectrograph in speech disorders has been its application in studying the dysarthrias. In an exhaustive study, Lehiste (1965) applied spectrographic analyses to the speech of ten dysarthrics. Unfortunately, space does not allow for a review of this classic monograph here. Students of dysarthria are encouraged to read the original study. Briefly, she found diversified patterns among dysarthrics with variation across duration, frequency and quality parameters. Since Lehiste's study a number of researchers have employed the spectrograph to analyse speech patterns of various subgroups of dysarthria in order to ascertain patterns which may be associated with lesion types. Spectrographic measures used to describe these patterns are discussed here.

Netsell and various colleagues have used spectrographic analysis as one adjunct to other physiological measures of dysarthria. These spectrographic observations have generally been concerned with dysarthria due to cerebellar lesions (ataxic dysarthrias). In a case study of an ataxic, Kent and Netsell (1975) observed that their subject's utterances were half again as long as that of their control subjects. While the ataxic's fundamental frequency generally had a monotonic contour, it also had marked upward and downward sweeps and instances of vocal fold aperiodicity. Normal VOT and frication durations were noted for /p, z/ and the syllabic nuclei of words were of normal duration. In another case study of paroxysmal dysarthria, Netsell and

Kent (1976) found long glide and syllable durations, weak or absent plosion of /t/, less prominent resonances and little shift in formant frequencies for /ri/. Kent, Netsell and Abbs (1979) analysed speech patterns in five individuals with cerebellar disease. Spectrographic analysis showed alterations in timing patterns with prolongation of a variety of segments and a tendency toward equalised syllable durations. Vowel formant structure was judged to be essentially normal except for transitional segments. Amount of duration lengthening appeared to be related to severity of the disorder. Fundamental frequency contours were monotonic or had a syllable-falling pattern.

Kent and Rosenbek (1982) studied prosodic parameters in Parkinsonian and right-hemisphere damaged dysarthrics. Spectrograms for the Parkinsonian dysarthrics were characterised by a lack of stop gaps, low intensity frication, reduced formants, antiresonance and continuous voicing. While some of the speakers had a normal or fast speaking rate, their articulators were not reaching their targets. Right-hemisphere lesioned subjects' spectrograms were characterised by reduction of acoustic energy in the midfrequency range, antiresonance and reduced acoustic contrast. Kent and Rosenbek noted the similarity between these two dysarthrias and labelled them as 'aprosodic'.

In a series of studies, Farmer and various colleagues analysed durational aspects of the speech of athetotic and spastic cerebral palsied speakers. Farmer *et al*. (1976) described a prevocalisation (PV) in athetotic speakers and its frequency of occurrence before various sounds in initial sentence and interspeech word sounds. PVs occurred more often before sounds requiring precise coordination of speech musculature and were positively related to other speech duration measures. In a follow-up study, Farmer and Lencione (1977) analysed PV occurrence in athetotic and spastic speakers. They found that athetoids used PVs significantly more frequently than did spastics, and the PVs used by the athetoids were significantly longer than those used by the spastics. VOTs were analysed in athetotic speakers (Farmer, 1977) and were found to be generally longer than those used by normal speakers. Further, each subject showed widely different but individually consistent VOT modes. When PVs occurred before stops, they appeared more frequently and were of longer duration before the voiced VOTs. VOTs were compared between athetotic and spastic speakers (Farmer, 1980) and while both groups had VOTs which were generally longer than those of normal speakers, the athetotic subjects had longer and more variable VOTs than did the spastic speakers.

Hearing Impaired

Another clinical population with poor intelligibility due to a range of speech mechanism involvements is the severely hearing impaired or deaf. Spectrographic studies have shown that this population's speech problems involve duration, frequency and quality parameters.

Gilbert and Campbell (1978) compared VOT between hearing impaired and control subjects. They found that voiceless VOTs were shorter in the speech of the hearing impaired, while voiced VOTs varied. They concluded that the hearing-impaired speakers did not differentiate between voiced and voiceless stop consonants or between stressed and unstressed contexts as did normally hearing speakers. VD was analysed in the speech of deaf children by Monsen (1974). He found that /i and I/ had more restricted durational ranges in the deaf than in normal speakers. Angelocci, Kopp and Holbrook (1964) analysed vowel formants in the speech of eleven-to-fourteen year old deaf and normally hearing boys. They found that the deaf had higher mean ranges of Fos and amplitude than did the normal hearing subjects. The mean ranges of the first three formants and amplitudes were, however, greater for the hearing than deaf subjects.

Voice Disorders

A classic study by Yanagihara (1967a) concerned spectrographic analysis of hoarseness. He found that hoarseness could be categorised into four types based on severity, and that these types perceptually positively correlated with hoarseness type as defined by the spectrographic analysis. The three acoustic parameters which define hoarseness include: (1) noise components in the main formants of each vowel; (2) high frequency noise components about 3,000 Hz, and (3) the loss of high frequency harmonic components. As severity of hoarseness increases, these components become exaggerated. Iwota and von Leden (1970) employed contour spectrography (distribution of acoustic energy which is usually represented by shades of black and grey to represent strong to weak intensity, respectively, at different frequency levels) with Yanagihara's (1967a) four types and found that this provided additional assessment data. Cooper (1974) also used Yanagihara's (1967a) four types to assess hoarseness in a large population. He found that most of these patients were using a too low Fo.

Two types of spastic dysphonia were spectrographically analysed by Wolfe and Bacon (1976). One subject's voice was spectrographically characterised by a breakdown in formant structure with the addition of fricative fill (or the vertical striations falling between resonance bars which has been associated with breathy voice quality) superimposed upon resonance bars. Spectrographic analysis of the second subject was characterised by widely and irregularly spaced vertical striations. Wolfe and Bacon noted that while acoustic analysis revealed two patterns, direct physiological assessment was needed to understand the underlying physical differences. VOT in oesophogeal speakers was analysed by Christensen, Weinberg and Alfonso (1978). They found that while these speakers were able to maintain the voice-voiceless contrast, the oesophogeal speakers' VOTs were shorter than those of normal speakers.

Aphasia and Apraxia

A recent application of spectrography has been in the area of aphasia and apraxia. The issue of whether or not apraxia is primarily an inability to programme articulators or involves linguistic preprogramming dysfunction was addressed by Collins, Rosenbek and Wertz (1978). By comparing VD and word durations of increasingly complex linguistic stimuli (jab, jabber, jabbering) they were able to determine that apraxics did decrease the primary vowel duration as the word lengthened. This indicated that apraxics do retain linguistic competence. However, both VD and word durations were longer in apraxic speech indicating that their primary problem was at the level of programming for articulation.

Several studies (Blumstein *et al.*, 1977, 1980; Freeman, Sands and Harris, 1978) have been concerned with VOT in apraxic and aphasic speakers. Blumstein *et al.* (1977) demonstrated that anterior aphasics could perceive the voice-voiceless phonetic contrast for alveolar stops, although their VOT productions included both phonetic and phonemic errors. Freeman *et al.* (1978) compared VOTs for voiced and voiceless stops in the speech of one apraxic subject. While his stops were all characterised by voicing lags, there were small differences between his voiced and voiceless sounds. In a larger study comparing Broca's and Wernicke's aphasics with control and dysarthric speakers, Blumstein *et al.* (1980) found that VOT further differentiated between phonemic and phonetic error differences. Control and Wernicke's subjects maintained definite voice-voiceless contrasts, while Broca's subjects showed marked overlay of VOT for voiced and voiceless productions. The dysarthric subject, by contrast, showed no phonetic overlap although his VOTs were quite varied in the voiceless range. These data led Blumstein *et al.* (1980) to conclude that Broca's aphasia reflects an articulatory coding rather than a low-level motor disorder.

A similar study analysing frication was done by Code and Ball

(1982). They found that vocal fold vibration was absent from voiced fricatives in a Broca's aphasic patient while vowel duration differences preceding fricatives was normally maintained. Further, they found that duration for voiced and voiceless fricatives was longer than that of normal speakers. They interpreted their results as supporting the notion that apraxia of speech constitutes a phonetic rather than a phonemic disorder. Code and Ball further suggested that different mechanisms may be involved in separate control of phonation and articulation.

More recently, Kent and Rosenbek (1982) compared prosody among several types of dysarthric and apraxic speakers. Their spectrographic observations of apraxic speech indicated prolongation of vowels (with stressing of normally unstressed vowels), inappropriate pause insertion and prolongation of transitions.

Although only recently applied to the study of aphasia and apraxia, spectrography has been of value in resolving theoretical issues as well as in assessing better methods of treatment.

Language Disorders

Another recent application of spectrography has been to study speech segment durations in language-disordered children. Based on the finding that speech segmental duration control is developmental in normal children (Tingley and Allen, 1975; Farmer and Florance, 1977) compared VOT, VD and VD relationships between language-disordered and control subjects matched for chronological age. While voiceless VOT and VD were generally longer and more variable in the language-disordered group, significance was found only for /æ/. Although VOT for /d/ was longer in the control group, it, as well as other VOTs and VDs were significantly more variable in the language-disordered group. When vowel lengthening rules were compared, 62.5 per cent of the language-disordered and 12.5 per cent of the control children violated one or more of these rules. In a follow-up study (Hambly and Farmer, 1982) VDs were compared between language-disordered children showing the open-syllable pattern and controls matched for age. Because of the simple (CVC) stimuli used, the open-syllable subjects were generally able to produce final sounds on the experimental task. However, the open-syllable children had significantly longer and more variable VDs than did their control group in the voiced consonant environment for words and phrases. While the voiceless stop consonant environment was also significantly different, the experimental group's VDs were only longer and more variable during single-word as opposed to phrase production. Bond and Wilson (1980) compared VOT in language-delayed and normal speaking children matched for language age. They found that the language-delayed children had more immature VOT patterns and used more prevoicing than did the control group.

Another group of children studied by Hellyer and Farmer (1982) were those who had been tracheotomised during babbling and normal controls matched for chronological age. Vowel formant relationships were compared for the two groups and no significant differences were found, leading the authors to conclude that babbling may not be necessary for later development of normal vowel production.

Clinical Application

As can be seen from the research, spectrography provides an extremely useful method for parameter analysis of speech and language disorders. Since the parameters of a disorder can be measured, one would expect that changes in these parameters brought about by treatment could also be documented using spectrography. This section will review studies which have been concerned with examining various clinical treatment results via spectrography.

Stuttering

A number of studies have shown that stutterers generally show shorter VDs and VOTs than do fluent speakers. One would expect then that successful treatment of stuttering would result in changes in these speech parameters. Metz *et al*. (1979b) compared VD and VOT in stutterers pre- and post-treatment. As well as showing an increase in fluency, their subject also demonstrated longer VDs and more voicing in stop consonant production post-treatment.

Dysarthrias

Spectrographic analysis has been used to examine the effects of treatment methods for dysarthric patients. Arnott *et al*. (1975) compared the speech of a patient with Steele-Olaewski-Richardson Syndrome before and after eight weeks of L-Dopa medication. Spectrographic and articulatory analyses revealed no effects for this treatment. Farmer and Green (1978) compared the speech of one spastic and two athetotic speakers under quiet and white noise side conditions. Word, interword and extraneous vocalisations varied across conditions for each speaker. Each speaker's response was individual with little significant change occurring in speaking durations. For these three speakers, auditory masking appeared to interfere with rather than enhance speech production. The negative results of these studies, while discouraging, are important in planning treatment programmes. Other treatment methods should be tested in this manner to ascertain if their hypothesised effect is affecting the speaking parameters intended.

Hearing-impaired

Spectrographic analysis was used by Wirz, Subtelny and Whitehead (1981) to compare vocal tension in deaf subjects before and after a period of treatment. They found acoustic abnormalities for pretreatment groups which suggested that deaf speakers were using a variety of physiological bases for vocal tension. While vocal tension was reduced in these speakers, Wirz *et al.* emphasised the need to differentiate the nature of the tension before planning the treatment programme. Since the speaking patterns of the severely hearing-impaired and deaf are so complex and varied, spectrographic analysis can provide added data for assessment. As shown in the Wirz *et al.* (1981) study, additional acoustic data may lead to differential treatment planning for this population.

Voice Disorders

A number of articles are available which demonstrate the use of spectrography in assessing vocal disorders before and after treatment. Rontal, Rontal and Rolnick (1975a) have summarised the acoustic characteristics of nodules, vocal cord paralysis and functional dysphonias, emphasising the value of spectrographic analysis. However, they note that since vocal disorders share similar acoustic characteristics, spectrography should be used in conjunction with indirect laryngoscopy. Kelman *et al.* (1981) found that while aerodynamic assessment could be rapidly carried out and provided objective numerical data, the spectrographic analysis provided additional and important information for assessment. Cooper (1974) found that most hoarse patients were using a too low Fo and after a treatment period designed to increase Fo, hoarseness was significantly decreased in these individuals and remained so after a follow-up period.

Spectrographic analysis has also been used to demonstrate the effectiveness of vocal cord injection in patients with vocal fold paralysis (Rontal, Rontal and Rolnick, 1975b; Reich and Lerman, 1978). Post-treatment acoustic analyses showed elimination of frication and aperiodicity as well as an increase in harmonic energy.

Aphasia and Apraxia

Spectrography has been used as an adjunct in planning treatment for aphasic patients. Freeman *et al*. (1978) confirmed the voicing disorder via spectrography which had been analysed phonetically by Sands, Freeman and Harris (1978). Laughlin, Naeser and Gordon (1979) varied Melodic Intonation Theraphy (MIT) stimuli by three syllable duration conditions and found that their subjects responded most accurately to syllables occurring two per second as opposed to less than one or one and a half per second. Such a finding provides specific information regarding the manner in which MIT should be presented.

Conclusion

As seen in the review of the literature, spectrography has widespread application across speech and language disorders. While it has been primarily used in diagnostics, an important application is the documentation of speech improvement due to clinical treatment. Based on its widespread application, a spectrograph should be a basic instrument in every speech and hearing clinic. However, availability of the spectrograph is generally limited to university, speech science laboratories and large hospital settings. This limiation exists for basically two reasons. First, the instrumentation is thought to be relatively expensive and, secondly, speech-language clinicians may not have been trained to use the instrumentation. Each of these situations can be easily resolved.

Cost of instrumentation is justified by the improvement that can be made in delivery and quality of services. The literature reviewed in this chapter provides strong support for the use of spectrography.

While all speech-language clinicians should have been trained in the use of spectrography, the fact is that this is not the case. While the onus of remediating this situation primarily rests with the universities, other measures may also be taken. Wider clinical use of spectrography could be made if clinicians could send audio taped samples of speech to centres where spectrograms could be made from them. Workshops concerning how to design speech stimuli, make quality recordings and analyse spectrograms, could be made available for participants. A small fee for this service could provide qualified graduate students additional fiscal support.

In summary, spectrography is a basic tool of speech-language science and should be a part of every treatment centre.

3 ELECTROMYOGRAPHY

Walter H. Moore, Jr.

Introduction to Electromyography

An Historical Overview

To the speech-language pathologist the application of electromyographic (EMG) procedures to the evaluation and treatment of speech-language disorders is relatively new; however, the study of muscles and muscle electricity is far from new. Basmajian's (1978) historic review reveals that muscles and their function were studied by such greats as Leonardo da Vinci and Andreas Vesalis (whose work 'Fabrica' has extended down to the present). At the end of the eighteenth century, it was Galvani who discovered that skeletal muscles would contract when stimulated electrically and that they produced a current when contracted. It was the Frenchman, Duchenne (1867), who applied Galvani's discoveries to the systematic study of skeletal muscles. Yet, it was not until the twentieth century that methods for detecting and measuring the minute electrical activity from muscles themselves became widely available (Basmajian, 1978).

With an increased sophistication in electronics after World War II, there was a corresponding increase in the improvement of electromyographic equipment and, consequently, EMG investigations. One of the most important early studies published leading to the general acceptance of EMG was conducted by Inman, Saunders, and Abbott (1944) who investigated the muscle movements of the shoulder region. It was during this time that EMG studies of the speech apparatus, particularly the intrinsic laryngeal muscles, began to emerge (for example, Feinstein, 1945-1946; Weddell, Feinstein, and Pattle, 1944) which have furthered our understanding of the correlations between laryngeal behaviour and voice production. Today EMG procedures have been used to investigate and treat a wide range of disorders including those which are stress-related (Stoyva, 1977), related to neuromuscular disorders (Inglis, Campbell and Donald, 1977) and those related to disorders of speech and language (to be reviewed below).

41

The Physiological Basis of Electromyography

Voluntary muscles are made up of many different and separate muscle fibres. These muscle fibres are arranged in parallel in some muscles, extending from one end of the muscle to the other. Other muscle fibres are short originating in one tendon and inserted into another tendon which runs the length of the muscle (Lippold, 1967). Muscle fibres, when contracted, can shorten to about 57 per cent of their resting length (Haines, 1932, 1934).

The basis for muscle contraction and thus the electrical activity term electromyography is the neuromuscular mechanism called the motor unit. As Cooper (1965) has described it, this mechanism is composed of a single neurone, located within the Central Nervous System (CNS), and a group of muscle fibres (as many as 200) to which it is connected by its motor endplates. The nerve cell body, the long axon, the terminal branches of the axon, and all the muscle fibres connected via the motor endplates comprise a motor unit. Whenever an impulse travels along the axon all of the muscle fibres in one motor unit contract almost simultaneously.

EMG activity is generated when an impulse travels down the axon to the myoneural junction or endplates and causes an action potential at the muscle fibres. This action potential is a wave of depolarisation (a temporary reversal of the polarisation of the cell membrane) that moves along the muscle fibre. Surface depolarisation precedes the contractile mechanism with the muscle fibres (Lippold, 1967). The depolarisation and contraction of the muscle fibres is seen as electrical activity. Electrical discharges of the muscle fibres are quite brief (median duration of 9 ms) and have an amplitude which is measured in microvolts (one microvolt is one-millionth of a volt) (Basmajian, 1978). When recording EMG with surface electrodes it is not unusual to record the electrical activity of many muscle fibres and motor units simultaneously. (Considerable research has been generated which addresses the physiological bases of EMG and the reader is referred to Harris (1981), Basmajian (1978), and Lippold (1967) for further discussion of these processes. A basic understanding is minimal to interpreting research in speech-language pathology using electromyographic procedures.)

Instrumentation Used in the Study of Electromyography

Electrodes. The first and perhaps most basic component is the electrode. Simply stated, the electrode connects the biological preparation or organism to an electrical instrument. While they are basic components their vulnerability and importance to recording cannot be overstressed.

The major concern with electrodes is *polarisation*. This process occurs when oppositely charged ions of the biological preparation are attracted to the respective electrode poles. An accumulation of ions at the electrodes affects the current and voltage being recorded and leads to errors. Because of this potential for error, nonpolarisable electrodes are recommended for electrophysiological research (for example, silver/silver chloride electrodes).

A second major concern with electrodes is their impedance with the biological preparation. If impedance (a measure of resistance across several frequencies relative to a reference) is high, the electrical signal being recorded will be erroneously reduced. This problem can, in part, be overcome by careful preparation of the area to which the electrodes are to be placed and proper connection of the electrodes to reduce the probability of high impedance. (The interested reader is referred to Cooper, Osselton, and Shaw (1974) for a complete discussion of electrodes.)

Generally three different types of electrodes are used in EMG recording: surface, needle, and hooked-wire electrodes. While needle and hooked-wire electrodes provide the 'cleanest' signal or recording from a single muscle, it is fairly common for surface electrodes to be used in biofeedback or treatment studies (Guitar, 1975; Moore, Cunko and Flowers, 1979). While surface electrodes provide a signal that may be influenced by several muscle groups, their use seems justified in clinical research and treatment due to the relative ease of application, reduced discomfort to the client, and non-invasive nature.

Amplifiers. Because the electrophysiological voltage associated with EMG activity is so small (measured in microvolts which are a millionth of a volt) it must be increased so that a measurable signal can be obtained. The function of the amplifier is to increase the voltage (within known calibration criteria) of a bioelectrical signal for display and processing purposes. The amplifier must be of sufficient quality to minimise distorting the actual bioelectrical signal when it is amplified. Special attention to total amplification and frequency response characteristics of an amplifier is important when conducting electrophysiological research (Camougis, 1970).

Read-out Devices. Once an electrical signal is amplified, to be useful, it must be displayed or recorded so that we may observe some parameter of its physical properties (for example, amplitude, frequency and/or duration). Typically, the EMG signal is displayed on a cathode ray oscilloscope (CRO) which can be seen on a cathode ray tube (CRT). One disadvantage to the CRT is that it has a limited time duration that can be displayed and 'hard copies' can be had only by photographing the displayed signal. To overcome this disadvantage ink-writing oscillographs are used that provide a permanent or hard copy on polygraph paper. (See Chapter 1 for further discussion of recording and storing techniques.)

Other devices used are integrators. These devices sample (average integrator) or continuously cumulate (cumulative integrator) the amplitude or energy associated with the EMG signal. Average or cumulative energy can also be displayed on a CRT or ink-writing oscillograph. The advantage of using an integrator is that pretreatment energy levels can more easily be compared to treatment levels for measurement purposes.

Figure 3.1: Typical Systems Set-up for Recording EMG and Providing Feedback

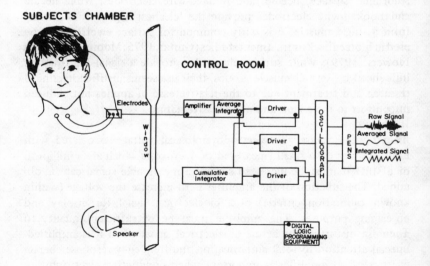

Today, it is becoming more commonplace for EMG laboratories to reduce and process electrophysiological data with micro-computers. Not only can computers be used to gather, store, display and retrieve data, they can also be used to analyse the frequency, amplitude and durational components of the signal. Obviously, micro-computers have reduced the time involved in processing and gathering electrophysiological data and elevated the entire process from mediocrity. With the cost of micro-computers becoming more reasonable, it is no longer necessary to record electrophysiological signals on FM tape-recorders for off-line processing. With today's technology, on-line processing of physiological signals is rapidly becoming the norm.

Figure 3.1 is a typical instrumentation system for recording raw, average integrated, and cumulative integrated EMG and providing the subject with feedback.

Research and Therapeutic Application of EMG to Speech-Language Disorders

When EMG is recorded for assessing muscle functions, the system shown in Figure 3.1 is typically used. Two electrodes are placed over the muscle to be assessed and a ground is placed on a nearby site on the subject's body. The electrodes are connected to the amplifier via an electrode cable. The signal is amplified and then displayed on a CRT, ink-writing oscillograph, or computer terminal. Preparation of the electrode site and placement of the electrode is a critical aspect of recording EMG. Poor preparation of the electrode site can result in high impedance which will reduce the biological signal. (Impedance should always be below 10k ohms. In most amplifiers 10k ohms of impedance will result in a 1 per cent reduction in the recorded signal.) If repeated measurements are to be made, as will be the case in treatment studies, exact electrode placement must be known so that the electrode can be replaced in exactly the same area for each measurement (standard electrode placements can be found in Lippold (1967) and Davis (1952)).

When EMG procedures are used in the clinical setting or in applied research, it is typically done using a biofeedback paradigm. These procedures provide the subject with auditory, visual, or a combination of auditory and visual feedback relative to the subject's EMG energy levels. Typically, the EMG signal from the amplifier is interfaced with a signal detection device such as a Schmitt trigger or a voltage comparator. These devices are then interfaced with frequency oscillators and amplifiers and/or lamp devices for providing feedback to the subject about the raw or integrated EMG energy.

Depending on the experimental design or the treatment programme, EMG data are first gathered without feedback to obtain a baseline level of energy. Following the gathering of baseline data, treatment sessions are begun which provide the subject with feedback to increase or decrease the amount of EMG activity. Many designs call for the withdrawal of treatment with a return to baseline where no feedback is provided to evaluate the treatment effects with a subsequent return to treatment to re-establish the treatment effects. This is referred to as an ABAB design where A = baseline and B = treatment. The importance of this kind of design is that it allows for the establishment of a reliable and valid treatment effect which can be observed in the withdrawal and re-establishment phases of the programme or design.

While the application of EMG biofeedback has not been extensive in speech-language pathology to date, those studies that have been reported provide convincing evidence for the remediation and modification of a variety of speech-language disorders. The discussion that follows will provide some of the research and therapeutic application of EMG procedures to the understanding and treatment of speech-language disorders.

Voice and Voice Disorders

The larynx may be viewed as having two discrete and important functions (Basmajian, 1978). The first and perhaps most basic is concerned with respiration, protection of the pulmonary apparatus, and trapping air in the thoracic cavity, allowing a build-up of pressure, to support the upper extremities during lifting. These activities are accomplished by the valve- or sphincteric-like functions of the vocal folds. The second function is that of phonation or sound production.

The neurochronaxic theory of phonation advanced by Husson (1950), and supported by Portmann (1957) suggested that the electromyographic oscillations of the vocal folds had the same frequency as the emitted sound. Thus, pitch or frequency was regarded as representing the direct vibrations of the vocal folds.

While the neurochronaxic explanation for voice production was widely rejected (for example, Rubin, 1960; Spoor and Van Dishoeck, 1960) it was the work of Faaberg-Andersen (1957) which provided convincing evidence failing to support Husson's theory. Inserting needle electrodes into the cricothyroid, vocalis, arytenoiderus, thyroarytenoid, and posterior cricoarytenoid muscles he recorded EMG activity and phonation simultaneously on a tape recorder.

Faaberg-Andersen found that at rest there was only a slight activity in the adductors contrasted with the abductors which were quite active. During phonation an increase in electrical activity for the cricothyroid, thyroarytenoid, vocalis, lateral cricoarytenoid, and arytenoid muscles (the adductors) was found (Faaberg-Andersen, 1957, 1964). Interestingly, maximum activity was seen before an audible tone was recorded. While activity decreases with an audible tone it remains greater than at rest. Corresponding typically with the cessation of the audible tone is the cessation of increased electrical activity. Failing to support the neurochronaxic theory of voice production, Faaberg-Andersen did not observe an increase in EMG activity of the adductor muscles with increasing pitch. According to Basmajian (1978):

> Thus Faaberg-Andersen does not support the theory that the frequency of vibration of the vocal cords during phonation of a tone changes directly with the frequency of nerve impulses and contractions of the muscle fibres. Faaberg-Andersen upholds the orthodox view that the vibrations of the vocal cord are passive and independent of the frequency of motor unit contractions. (p. 373)

Numerous investigations have been conducted on the regulation of pitch. Investigations by Hirano, Vennard and Ohala (1970), Shipp and McClone (1971), Gay *et al.* (1972) and Baer, Gay and Niimi (1976) have all shown increased activity of the cricothyroid with increases in pitch which is consistent with the function of this muscle in lengthening (thus reducing mass) the vocal folds. An increase in the activity of the thyroarytenoids during increases in pitch has also been reported.

While only a brief summary of some of the functions of the laryngeal muscles have been provided, these studies do suggest that EMG activity associated with pitch changes seems to function to change the physical characteristics of the vocal folds (lengthening, shortening, etc.) which, consequently, change their vibratory characteristics. Thus the activity is related, in most cases, to vibratory characteristics and not the vibration of the folds *per se*. These findings are in support of the myoelastic-aerodynamic theory which states that the vocal folds are set into vibration by the air stream from the lungs and trachea. The vibratory frequency of the folds is dependent upon their length in relation to tension and mass which is effected by the intrinsic laryngeal muscles.

Hyperfunction has been described by Froeschels (1943) as the excessive use of muscular force in the vocal tract. Hyperfunctional use of the vocal mechanism has been regarded as the primary cause of pathological and functional voice disorders (Brodnitz, 1965). Data reported by Hirano, Koike and Joyner (1969) has indicated that hyperfunctional voice disorders can be accompanied by increased activity of the cricothyroid, lateral cricoarytenoid, vocalis, and sternohyoid muscles. These reports would support the notion that reduced hyper-tinesity in the laryngeal area would accompany an improvement in hyperfunctional voice disorders and provide a rationale for the application of EMG biofeedback procedures in their treatment. Additionally, the evaluation of a hyperfunctional voice disorder is often limited to a perceptual analysis of the auditory characteristics because the laryngeal structures are inaccessible. While instrumentation is available for some of the acoustical analyses the majority is still dependent upon the perceptions of the clinician. EMG and biofeedback procedures can be helpful with this problem to some extent by recording the muscle activity in the laryngeal area and relating it to the subject's laryngeal tension (Prosek *et al.*, 1978; Lyndes, 1975).

Lyndes (1975) has reported the use of a biofeedback procedure in functional dysphonia. Criteria for the use of biofeedback has been (1) resistance of the vocal problem to standard techniques and (2) a demonstrated vocal problem for over a year prior to the initiation of EMG biofeedback procedures (no rationale was given for the criteria). While many investigations have used the frontalis muscle in general relaxation studies, Lyndes has found the sternohyoid muscle more sensitive to laryngeal activity. The subjects are first trained in general relaxation, without vocal production, using auditory and visual feedback. During sessions where training is given with phonation only visual feedback is provided so that the subject can better attend to his/her voice without the interference of auditory feedback which was reported to be distracting. While Lyndes indicated that his use of biofeedback has been successful in the treatment of several patients with voice problems no data are provided that support his claims. Yet, he does provide a treatment procedure that could easily be adopted in the treatment of voice disorders.

Perhaps the most extensive research reporting on the efficacy of EMG biofeedback in the treatment of hyperfunctional voice disorders is that of Prosek *et al.* (1978). In their investigation six subjects who produced speech with excessive laryngeal tension participated in 14 30-minute biofeedback sessions. Two of their patients had vocal nodules, one had contact ulcers, one a small carcinoma removed from one vocal fold, one recurrent traumatic laryngitis and the sixth spastic dysphonia. For each subject EMG was measured with bipolar surface electrodes placed over the cricothyroid region. This site was chosen after pilot studies had shown EMG activity during phonation and during approximation of the vocal folds without phonation. The amplified, average integrated signal was used to control the output of a voltage controlled oscillator and a noise generator. When the EMG energy was below a preselected threshold, the voltage controlled oscillator was activated driving a pure tone which increased or decreased as the integrator energy increased or decreased. The noise generator was activated when the subject's energy levels surpassed the preselected threshold levels. The amplified signals from the oscillator and noise generator were outputed to the subject's earphones in a sound-treated room. A progressive shaping procedure was used systematically to reduce muscle activity. When the subject was able to keep the EMG activity below threshold 80 per cent of the time during a speech task, the threshold was reduced by 5 mv. In addition to the EMG data, judgments of voice quality were obtained pre- and post-treatment by six speech-language pathologists.

Results from this investigation indicated that a subject with contact ulcers, a subject with traumatic laryngitis, and a subject with bilateral vocal nodules, who were able to reduce laryngeal EMG activity during speech production tasks, showed a corresponding improvement in voice quality. In fact, a subsequent laryngeal examination of the subject with contact ulcers revealed that they were no longer present and the subject with traumatic laryngitis had not experienced any hoarseness or aphonia following training and demonstrated generalisation of the EMG treatment effects two, four, and eight weeks after the final training session! The third subject with bilateral vocal nodules showed inconsistent generalisation of improved voice quality in situations remote from the training or clinical environment indicating greater stimulus control of her behaviour to the training environment. The three subjects that did not demonstrate improvement in vocal behaviour and/or decreased EMG activity were those that had a neurogenic disorder and a poor prognosis for recovery (spastic dysphonia) or those that had structural damage (surgical removal of vocal nodules and surgical removal of a carcinoma with extensive radiation therapy).

The importance of the Prosek *et al* . (1978) investigation is that it provided clear empirical evidence for the usefulness of EMG biofeedback procedures in cases of demonstrated hyperfunction as the underlying aetiology of voice disorders and shows the reversibility of a pathological condition (contact ulcers) associated with vocal hyperfunction. Important also was the finding that treatment effects and improved vocal behaviour could be generalised to situations remote from the training environment and in follow-up sessions where no biofeedback treatment was provided. Additionally, it reveals, as would be expected, that EMG biofeedback procedures are not as effective in those cases where the vocal disorder is a result of structural damage or change.

The credibility of this investigation and the validity of the results is enhanced through their application of carefully designed and controlled experimental/clinical procedures and is a reflection of the quality of results that can be expected when good procedures are used in the management of hyperfunctional voice disorders and pathologies. This investigation can well serve as a procedural model for the application of EMG biofeedback in the remediation of hyperfunctional voice disorders.

Neurological Disorders of Speech-language

Persons with neurological disorders of speech often have difficulties which are due to paralysis or paresis of the speech musculature. The term that is generally applied to speech disorders resulting from paralysis or paresis is dysarthria. As Bloodstein (1979) has noted, dysarthria is a name of a speech disorder and is not a kind of paralysis or neurologic disease. Among the aetiologies of dysarthria are cerebral palsy, bulbar palsy, pseudobulbar palsy, Parkinsonism, chorea, multiple sclerosis, dystonia, and cerebrovascular accidents. The symptoms of dysarthria include consistently distorted articulation, slow-monotonous rate of speech, disturbances of speech rhythm or prosody and breathy or nasal voice quality, which may also have a strangled or strained quality. This symptomotology results from paralysis or paresis of the muscles for breathing, phonation, resonation, and articulation (Bloodstein, 1979).

To appreciate the motor disturbances associated with dysarthria it is necessary to have a basic understanding of the neural basis of a motor nerve pathway. Generally, if we perform a voluntary motor act, a motor nerve pathway in the central nervous system (CNS), which comprises the brain and spinal cord, must first direct nerve impulses from the brain to the spinal cord. Impulses for different muscles terminate at points along the spinal cord. At these points of termination the motor pathway in the peripheral nervous system (the system which connects the CNS to other parts of the body) directs the impulses to the appropriate muscle via its motor unit. Neurones which send impulses within the CNS are called upper motor neurones, while those in the peripheral nervous system are called lower motor neurones. Different muscular dysfunctions result from damage to various sites in the central and peripheral nervous system. A full discussion of these speech characteristics and the neuro-mechanisms associated with them may be found in Darley, Aronson, and Brown (1975).

Apraxia is also a disorder associated with impairment of motor speech movements. For years apraxia has been described as an inability to make articulatory movements or to programme such movements due to damage to the third frontal convolution of the left frontal lobe (Broca's area). However, recent evidence suggests that apraxia or kinesthetic motor aphasia can also result from damage to the somatic-sensory area of the parietal lobe posterior to the central fissure (Luria and Hutton, 1977). This would imply that the disorder results from a lack of kinesthetic feedback from the peripheral speech musculature. Support for this position has been provided by Rosenbek, Wertz and Darley (1973) who found apraxic subjects to be inferior to controls on tasks of oral form discrimination, two-point discrimination and mandibular kinesthesia, all of which depend on kinesthetic feedback. Results from Luria and Hutton (1977) and Rosenbek *et al.*'s (1973) investigations indicate that the disruption of internal feedback generated by the peripheral speech musculature is responsible for the motor speech disorders seen in apraxia. These observations would suggest that external muscle feedback might be helpful in overcoming apraxia disorders.

Non-fluent aphasia or motor aphasia is typically associated with cortical damage to the third frontal convolution of the left hemisphere. While this is the typical anatomical association with motor aphasia, Ojeman (1976) has shown that lesions in patients with motor aphasia often extend down into the subcortical areas to the pulvinar, an associative nucleus of the thalamus that connects anterior and posterior speech-language areas of the brain (Brown, 1975). The speech of non-fluent aphasics is characterised by a slow and laborious rate, hesitations, errors of articulation, and a marked reduction in grammatical structures referred to as agrammatism.

Perhaps due to the nature of aphasia, there is a paucity of research and clinical articles that have applied EMG procedures to understanding and modification of the speech-language disorders of the aphasic patient. By far the greatest application of EMG procedures with stroke patients has been in the area of footdrop, reduced hand function, and shoulder subluxation in an effort for the patient to discover and use motor pathways that have not been damaged and have been dormant (Basmajian, 1981). While the research is limited in the area of aphasia and EMG, that which has been reported does pave the way for both the need and the directions for future research.

Shankweiler, Harris and Taylor (1968) investigated the electromyographic pattern associated with the articulation of motor aphasia. Their five adult subjects ranging in age from 39 to 61 years of age had vascular lesions involving the anterior portions of the left cerebral hemisphere. Each had right hemiparesis and severe expressive aphasia with preservation of comprehension. The authors reported that at the time of testing the aphasic symptoms were 'greatly diminished,' leaving the articulatory deficit as the major impairment (this would suggest that their subjects may have been apraxic or dysarthric as defined above). After placing surface electrodes on three locations of the lips and tongue and one under the chin, subjects were allowed to adapt to speaking with the electrodes in place. Electromyograms were recorded while the subjects repeated one-syllable words and were compared to those recorded from normal speakers. Results from the aphasic subjects revealed grossly abnormal patterns, great variability in the timing of sequential movements, prolonged and variable duration for vowels, labial consonants in the initial position were more defective than those in the terminal position, and peaks from the electrode placements revealed a reduction in the ability to execute independent movements of the articulators. Shankweiler *et al.*'s (1968) investigation provided important information about the temporal and spatial organisation of defective speech which they state could not have been obtained with procedures which analyse only the acoustic parameters of speech. Results from this investigation reinforce the use of electromyography in assessing both the temporal and spatial characteristics of speech disorders which have a motor programming deficit component. Inferentially these results suggest that EMG procedures could be used to assess the effectiveness of rehabilitation training programmes aimed at these parameters by comparing pre- and post-treatment electromyograms. Additionally, it is quite conceivable that external feedback associated with the activity of the speech musculature could improve both the temporal and spatial components of the aphasic's speech (an inference which is supported in an investigation with apraxic patients reported below).

Huffman (1978) in a preliminary study of EMG biofeedback treatment of orofacial dysfunction of patients suffering from hemiparesis or quadriparesis resulting from vascular lesions with unilateral neglect and apraxia compared the effectiveness of electromyographic biofeedback and mirror (visual) feedback. Two of her patients received mirror feedback only while two other matched patients received mirror feedback for the first week and added EMG feedback to the visual training the second week. Four categories of oral motion were investigated: lip approximation, puckering, and sucking and blowing on a straw. Results showed EMG biofeedback training to be more efficient and more 'functionally effective' than the mirror or visual feedback conditions. Data obtained from the patients in the EMG condition for the oral tasks indicated complete volitional control and strength of motions for each task. Huffman suggested that EMG biofeedback is a means of externally providing information that is needed to complete the impaired interval feedback loop.

Huffman's findings with her apraxic patients are important for at least two reasons. Firstly, and perhaps most important, is the observation that EMG feedback has clinical utility in the management of apraxic patients. As she indicated her apraxic patients were able to gain volitional control for each of the oral tasks investigated as a result of an external substitute for proprioceptive loss. Secondly, her findings support the more recent explanation of apraxia of speech as an afferent-sensory disorder as opposed to an efferent-motor disorder of speech.

In the area of neurological disorders of speech-language the disorder of dysarthria, with its more obvious neuromuscular component, has been more vigorously investigated than other neurological disorders. Typically, the results from clinical investigations using EMG procedures with dysarthria have been very productive in demonstrating their usefulness in managing some of the disorder's symptoms.

Among the first to apply EMG biofeedback to a dysarthric speaker were Netsell and Cleeland (1973). Their dysarthric Parkinsonian patient demonstrated hypertonicity of the lips to such a degree that it resulted in complete bilateral contraction. Using a programme designed to reduce EMG activity associated with lip hypertonia they were successful in showing complete retraction of the lips bilaterally. These results were obtained after five half-hour sessions. Treatment effects were also demonstrated during speech although some retraction continued to be seen.

In a more extensive study which investigated the effects of EMG biofeedback in a Parkinsonism patient who exhibited lip hypertonia and retraction, Hand, Barns and Ireland (1979) provided feedback during a non-speech programme and a speech programme incorporating five speech tasks of increasing complexity and assumed difficulty. An important finding of this investigation was that the subject was able to reduce the level of muscular activity when presented with feedback in both the non-speech and the speech tasks. The authors also found a decrease in muscular EMG activity over the six sessions during instructions to contract. They attributed this finding to the patient's relearning agonistic-antagonistic muscle control with a corresponding decrease in simultaneous contractions (Leanderson, Persson and Ohman, 1970).

While the above investigations appear to indicate the effectiveness of biofeedback procedures in decreasing EMG activity the experimental design employed in some do not allow us to address the issue of effectiveness of the procedures. The lack of baseline data preceding the application of biofeedback training in some of the studies greatly reduces our ability to determine if EMG activity would have decreased in the experimental situation without feedback (the well known and very real 'placebo effect'). We are also provided with little data on the effects of such training on the patients actual speech behaviour. While, for example, the Hand *et al.* (1979) investigation explores different speech tasks during conditions of EMG biofeedback, no reports of pre- and post-treatment speech evaluations were provided. Indeed, the application of EMG biofeedback procedures to speech-language disordered patients requires explanation of not only electrophysiological data but also the corresponding behavioural data in carefully controlled research and/or clinical designs. The reduction or increase in EMG activity via biofeedback procedures in-and-of itself does not justify their use with speech-language disordered persons unless a corresponding change in speech-language behaviour can be demonstrated. Failure to provide behavioural data that correponds to physiological data does not allow one to address the validity of the procedures in the rehabilitation of speech-language disorders.

Finley *et al.* (1976) investigated the effects of frontalis muscle biofeedback training on speech and motor tasks in six athetoid cerebral palsy patients. Prior to treatment each subject was evaluated for various speech and motor functions and re-evaluated on these same measures following treatment. Results of the investigation revealed reductions in frontalis EMG over the six-week course of training; there was also an improvement in both speech and motor functions when pre- and post-treatment scores were compared.

Finley *et al.* (1976) hypothesised that sensory feedback from the frontalis muscle leads to generalised relaxation resulting in reduction of stretch from the receptors of the gamma efferent systems which lead to increased internal feedback from intrafusal muscle spindle receptors. Thus, the indirect connection between speech and other motor behaviours with biofeedback of the frontalis muscle was accomplished by a 'spill-over' effect of increased internal feedback.

While the association between speech improvement and reduced frontalis activity appeared quite clear when pre- and post-treatment scores were compared, Finley *et al*. point out that they did not employ a no-treatment control group and, consequently, a practice effect could not conclusively be ruled out. Thus, in a systematic replication of this study, Finley *et al*. (1977) not only manipulated other independent variables, they employed a 'reversal' ABAB design which allowed them to observe increases and decreases in both EMG frontalis activity and speech/motor behaviour. In this investigation four spastic cerebral palsy children participated in frontalis EMG biofeedback training and speech and motor evaluations. Unlike the first investigation in which auditory feedback only was provided (clicks) in their second study both auditory (clicks) and visual (pen deflections of a micro-ampere meter) feedback was provided. Additionally, if subjects were successful in remaining below an established cumulative voltage threshold, they were provided with tangible positive reinforcement on an initial continuous reinforcement schedule which was gradually modified to an 80 per cent variable ratio schedule.

In the first baseline session EMG and speech/motor evaluations were recorded without biofeedback (A_1). During the first treatment phase (B_1), in which biofeedback was given, frontalis EMG decreased significantly with a corresponding improvement in speech and motor skills. Following a six week withdrawal of biofeedback treatment (A_2) an increase in EMG voltage and deterioration of speech and motor function was observed. Reinstatement of frontalis EMG biofeedback produced reacquisition of low frontalis EMG and recovery of speech and motor functions (B_2).

Finley *et al*'s (1977) application of an ABAB experimental design allows for conclusive statements to be made with regard to reduced frontalis EMG activity and speech/motor improvement. A clear relationship between these two independent variables was established with their four cerebral palsied patients. Not only is their study an excellent example of the application of reversal methods, it also provides us with an example of the use of a reinforcement paradigm, with the use of tangible reinforcement, and schedules of reinforcement in EMG biofeedback research with speech-language disordered patients.

Fluency or Stuttering Disorders

Disorders of fluency or stuttering have perhaps received the greatest attention by researchers exploring EMG correlates of disordered speech-language behaviour. The reason for this seems to be the obvious excessive muscle tension which often accompanies stuttering, particularly in the adult, and often thought to be the underlying cause of the disorder. Consequently, a considerable amount of research has been conducted of both a basic and applied nature over the years to understand the aetiology of stuttering, from a theoretical and descriptive perspective, and to develop treatment approaches aimed at the reduction of muscle tension.

The earliest suggestion that stuttering may be the result of a neuromuscular disorder was provided by Travis (1931) who hypothesised that stuttering is characterised by the asynchronous arrival of nerve impulses in the bilaterally paired jaw muscles. In 1934 Travis presented electromyographic data recorded from the left and right masseter muscles of 24 adult stutterers and non-stutterers. Travis reported that action potentials from the normal subjects were 'practically identical' while those from his stuttering subjects were described as 'strikingly different'. Other investigations reported at this time concerned with electromyography and stutterers (Strother, 1935; Morley, 1935; Steer, 1937) seemed generally to support Travis' findings which were interpreted as demonstrating a basic neurophysiological difference between stutterers and non-stutterers.

Williams (1955), however, failed to support the interpretation of differences in EMG patterns between stutterers and non-stutterers as indicating a basic neurophysiological difference between the two groups. In fact his findings, recorded from the masseter with surface electrodes, failed to find significant differences with regard to bilateral amplitude and the appearance of action potentials between the two sides of the jaw. Differences that were found between the two groups' EMGs were attributed to the excessive muscular tension and different patterns of jaw movement that typically accompanies stuttering.

A somewhat similar finding to that of Williams (1955) has recently been reported by Code (1979) who reported significant durational and amplitude measures between genuine and artificial stuttering using EMG procedures. The difference reported by Code appeared to be related to greater muscular tension in his stutterer as compared to his normal subject under conditions of delayed auditory feedback. Bar, Singer and Feldman (1969) have also found increased EMG in stutterers' laryngeal activity immediately preceding and during a stuttered response. A related finding has been reported by Metz, Conture and Colton (1976). In their investigation of temporal relations between the respiratory and laryngeal systems prior to stuttered dysfluencies they found a delay in laryngeal activities when measured with EMG procedures. It may well be that the excessive laryngeal tension that has been observed prior to and during stuttering has the general effect of 'slowing down' laryngeal transitions, therefore, the delay in laryngeal activity prior to stuttering reported by Metz *et al.* (1976) may be an artifact of excessive laryngeal tension.

In an extensive investigation using simultaneous recordings from the five intrinsic laryngeal muscles (posterior cricoarytenoid, interarytenoid, cricothyroid, thyroarytenoid and lateral cricoarytenoid), with an indwelling hook-wire electrode procedure, Freeman and Ushijima (1978) studied fluent and stuttered utterances in four stutterers with EMG. Results of their study revealed increased laryngeal activity during stuttering which was '. . . significantly higher than those levels necessary to produce the desired phonatory adjustments and vocal tract shape changes for the segmental content of the experimental passage.' (p. 556-557). (Their finding of a segmental component fits well with Moore and Haynes' (1980) segmentation dysfunction hypothesis as an aetiological factor in stuttering.) Freeman and Ushijima (1978) interpreted their findings as indicating a disruption of the reciprocity between abductor and adductor muscle groups which lead to laryngeal activities which are counterproductive to normal phonation and present their results as evidence of a laryngeal component in stuttering.

In two separate investigations Moore and his associates (Moore, Cunko and Flowers, 1979; Moore, Flowers and Cunko, 1981) investigated the relationships between electromyographic activity of selected speech-related muscle groups and dysfluencies during massed oral readings in non-stutterers and stutterers. Recordings from masseter and laryngeal groups in non-stutterers were gathered during five massed oral readings of the same 130-word passage. Results revealed a decrease in dysfluencies over the five trials and a significant decrease in EMG activity across trials for the laryngeal, but not the masseter site. Moore *et al.* (1979) interpreted these findings as providing support that changes in vocal behaviour occur during adaptation and are reflected in EMG activity. Continuing with this research approach, Moore *et al.* (1981) investigated EMG activity and dysfluencies in a group of stutterers using the same procedures. Interestingly, they did not replicate their findings with normally fluent subjects. Significant reductions in EMG activity and dysfluencies were not found for this group. However, EMG activity was shown to be related to the subjects' dysfluency

patterns over trials. Results showed moderate-to-high positive correlations for EMG activity and dysfluency. The authors interpreted
their results as indicating that dysfluency and modifications in overt
behaviours and oral musculature, reflected in EMG activity, are simultaneous occurrences.

The above investigations demonstrate some rather consistent relationships between EMG activity and the stuttered verbal behaviour of
stuttering individuals. These studies can provide a rationale for the
application of EMG biofeedback procedures in the clinical management of stuttering. The studies which follow illustrate the application
and findings from such procedures in stuttering management/thera-
peutics.

Guitar (1975) demonstrated decreased EMG activity over four
muscle groups (orbicularis oris superior, anterior belly of the digastric,
laryngeal site above the thyroid cartilage, frontalis muscle) when subjects were presented with an audio feedback signal. Subjects were
trained to reduce muscle activity prior to uttering sentences from a
list. Three subjects demonstrated different effects of the training:
one showed the greatest decrease in stuttering when muscle relaxation
occurred at the lip site; a second, the greatest reduction with muscle
activity reduction at the laryngeal site; while the third showed the
greatest decrease in stuttering with both lip and laryngeal site training.
Applying these EMG biofeedback procedures in the treatment of a
single subject's conversational speech also proved effective. For the
treatment programme, Guitar's subject was trained to reduce muscle
activity at the chin (determined to be the optimal site for treatment
by comparison of pre-utterance muscle action potential levels) and in
the following treatment sessions instructed to reduce muscle activity
before he uttered a word he thought he might stutter on. Afterward,
the subject relied on his own perceptions of his levels of chin EMG
activity. Treatment demonstrated a dramatic decrease in the frequency
of stuttering and generalisation of the treatment effect was shown in
a five-week follow-up session.

Employing similar procedures Lanyon, Barrington and Newman
(1976) investigated the effects of visual feedback on the reduction of
chin and masseter activity. Similar to Guitar's procedure, subjects were
first taught to reduce muscle activity by monitoring either an oscilloscope wave pattern or a modified voltmeter. Speech tasks involved
counting numbers and forming words during procedure one. During
their second procedure where subjects monitored a modified voltage
meter, subjects progress in a systematic sequence from one-syllable

words to four-syllable sentences. Results showed virtual elimination of stuttering during feedback with generalisation of the treatment effects during no-feedback trials.

Using a tone which increased in frequency in proportion to the amplitude of EMG activity Hanna, Wilfling and McNeill (1975) provided a stuttering subject with laryngeal feedback during speech tasks when he was instructed to produce a low-frequency tone. Results showed stuttering was reduced to less than 50 per cent of baseline during biofeedback conditions. Importantly, the subject was also provided with 'fake' feedback to determine if the reduction could be attributed to 'placebo' or masking factors. Results showed false feedback to be substantially less effective than genuine feedback which addresses the validity of the EMG biofeedback procedures. (The addition of the false feedback condition provides us with procedural evidences of the effectiveness of EMG biofeedback procedures in the reduction of stuttered verbal behaviour and the relationship between EMG activity, at selected speech-related sites, and stuttering.)

The final investigation to be reviewed using EMG biofeedback procedures with stutterers is that of Moore (1978). While this investigation also showed reductions in stuttering when auditory feedback was provided to stutterers associated with masseter or chin activity, it is different in that feedback was provided during a speech task rather than preceding it. Subjects were also provided discrete feedback in a progressive manner, that is, as subjects were able to meet criteria EMG levels, the threshold was made progressively lower until a point was reached when the tone could not be kept off at least 50 per cent of the time. Additionally, similar to the Lanyon *et al*. (1976) study, subjects progressed from relatively simple to increasingly more difficult tasks. Because this investigation used ABAB or ABA single subject designs, generalisations of the treatment effects could be assessed. All three subjects showed clinically significant decreases in dysfluencies and generalisations of the treatment effects for an oral reading task, while one of the subjects showed these effects for a conversational speech task as well. According to Moore, his subjects' strategies for manipulating the feedback tone seemed to be related to reductions in many of the motoric and prosodic complexities of speech. That is, there was not simply a reduction in EMG activity, but a change in vocal behaviour which seemed importantly involved in EMG amplitude decreases and enhanced fluency (a finding seen with many fluency enhancing methods).

The above investigations have shown dysfluencies to be reduced or eliminated when subjects are provided with feedback to reduce EMG activity in speech-related muscle groups. When viewed in concert with those investigations that have explored muscle activity and dysfluency, a rather clear relationship seems to emerge between dysfluencies and speech-related EMG activity. Yet, the reader is cautioned from seeing a simple relationship between EMG activity and dysfluency. It seems more likely that reductions in both dysfluencies and EMG activity is the outcome of a process and not the process itself. That is, subjects appear to develop vocal strategies (resulting in changes in vocal behaviours such as pitch, intensity, onset, rate, etc.) that are associated with reduced levels of EMG activity. It is often these very vocal changes that are responsible for reductions in dysfluency and not simply reduced muscle activity. When subjects or clients fail to reduce dysfluencies or decrease muscle activity, it may be a reflection of our failure to recognise these acts as the outcome of more subtle behavioural processes.

Conclusion

An understanding of the physiological basis of electromyography is clearly important for understanding speech and vocal behaviours. Not only do we benefit in our understanding of the nature of physiological aspects of normal speech production, but such knowledge can be applied to the speech and language disorders that have direct motor involvement or to those disorders that are the result of disrupted afferent feedback.

While our knowledge and the application of EMG, as related to speech and language disorders, has increased greatly during the past two or three decades, it is still apparent that EMG methodology and application is not a common procedure utilised by most speech-language pathologists. Yet, while the data are not all in, it is apparent from the studies reviewed that EMG procedures have a definite place in the assessment and management of speech and language disorders. The success of EMG biofeedback procedures in voice disorders, neurological disorders of speech-language, and stuttering is indeed impressive. While the instrumentation and procedures appear to be complicated and sophisticated for clinical application, their success in remediating a variety of speech and language disorders warrants their serious consideration, not only in the research laboratory but the clinical environment as well. Too, relatively inexpensive EMG biofeedback devices are readily available today which can be quite easily adapted for clinical purposes by the speech-language pathologist.

While the application of EMG procedures to speech and language disorders seems apparent, it is equally apparent that investigations into their use and application must continue. Procedures for the clinical application of EMG methodology need to be continually refined as do clinical and experimental designs for testing and demonstrating their validity. Indeed, the clinical application of EMG technology is not a simple task and we must realise that the results we obtain with this technology are only as good as the treatment and research procedures and designs that are used. Thoughtful and knowledgeable application has and will continue to be of benefit to persons with speech and language disorders.

4   ELECTROLARYNGOGRAPHY

Evelyn Abberton and Adrian Fourcin

Introduction

It is of considerable theoretical interest and practical value to be able to monitor, measure and display aspects of larynx activity in both normal and disordered speech. In this chapter we provide an introduction to a simple method of doing so that does not interfere with speech production.

Although an ordinary listener perceives speech as a whole, for the phonetician and speech pathologist it can be studied in terms of separate but interacting components from each of the points of view of speech production, acoustics and perception. Thus, in acoustic terms, the physical form of voiced speech (the most frequent and most energetic speech sounds) depends on a quasi-periodic sound source from the vibrating vocal folds in the larynx. This laryngeal tone, rich in harmonics, is called *voice*, and its production known as *phonation*; this component is filtered by the vocal tract due to the changing configurations and, therefore, resonances of the supra-glottal cavities produced by the movements and muscular tension of the articulators. Although phonation and resonance interact, the characteristics of each may be separated conceptually and experimentally, and one or the other may be selectively impaired. Thus, to consider two extreme conditions, in glossectomy, phonation and intonation are preserved, and in laryngectomy, although the normal source of speech is lost, articulatory capability is essentially intact.

From a perceptual point of view the laryngeal excitation components of speech are vitally related to both intelligibility and acceptability, through the segmental phonological voiced-voiceless contrast and through the non-segmental prosodic and paralinguistic systems of phonation type and tone and intonation: a speaker with the irregular and intermittent phonation and reduced fundamental frequency range associated with laryngitis is not so easily understood as when his larynx is adequately lubricated and vibrating normally. An adult male using falsetto voice is not so socially acceptable as his fellows with normal vocal fold vibration in an appropriate fundamental frequency range; and foreigners may err socially as well as linguistically when they use an inappropriate intonation pattern or phonation type. Type and rate of vocal fold vibration provide the essential skeleton of normal speech communication.

Type of vibration is responsible for vocal register; for a particular speaker a given vibration type (phonation type) is typically associated with a particular fundamental frequency range (Hollien, 1974). Rate of vibration (fundamental frequency) is the major correlate of the pitch patterns of the linguistic prosodic systems of tone and intonation. In tone languages (e.g. Chinese) the relative pitch height or contour with which a word is spoken changes the dictionary meaning of that word (Pike, 1948). The pitch patterns of intonation perform grammatical (prosodic) and attitudinal (paralinguistic) functions similar to those of punctuation in written language, but the number of contrasts involved is far greater. Relative pitch height, and direction and location of pitch changes need to be taken into account. It has been shown that both phonation type and fundamental frequency patterning contribute importantly to perceived voice quality (Abberton and Fourcin, 1978), normal individuals in age-, sex-, and accent-matched groups being easily identified even when no supraglottal resonance information is available. These experiments, with natural and synthetic stimuli, demonstrate the important indexical (speaker-identifying) role that laryngeal speech components play.

The importance of larynx activity as the framework for speech is also shown by the young child's early ability to perceive and produce the essential patterns of phonation and the basic tone and/or intonation contrasts of its native language well before segmental phonological contrasts and phonotactic patterning are controlled. It has frequently been observed that before the first birthday a child already shows language-specific intonation patterns, and Crystal (1975) reviewing the literature, suggests that by two and a half years of age the tone system of a tone language has been learned, and the major intonation contrasts in an intonation language. As yet there are hardly any reliable quantitative studies of this stage of language acquisition but an example of very early prosodic interaction between a mother and her baby has been studied by Fourcin (1978) using spectrographic techniques to measure the fundamental frequency contours and ranges of the mother's and baby's utterances during mutual imitation.

It is not surprising that larynx vibration pattern, fundamental frequency range and intonation are disordered in many speech pathologies, developmental and acquired, with a range of aetiologies. For example, laryngeal patterning problems may be associated with impaired hearing (Whetnall and Fry, 1964), emotional or psychiatric difficulties (Leff and Abberton, 1981; Greene, 1980) or hormonal imbalance (van Gelder, 1974), as well as those conditions with an obvious anatomical focus in the laryngeal assembly itself such as paralysis, inflammation, or growths benign or malignant. The voices of speakers with such conditions often pose considerable descriptive and therapeutic challenges, and electrolaryngography provides a convenient way of obtaining both qualitative and quantitative information on vocal fold vibration and its linguistic use, as well as providing a clinical tool for visual feedback therapy.

The Electrolaryngograph

The detailed patterns relating to, for example, laryngeal air velocity or glottal area variation as functions of time are not open to simple visual examination nor are their parameters available to the speaker on the basis of introspection as certain gross articulatory gestures are. Auditory analysis of intonation patterns is a skill that for many people is learned only after a painstaking apprenticeship. Several methods are available for examining vocal fold vibration but they all either depend on complex electronic processing of the acoustic speech signal or interfere with speech production (Fourcin and Abberton, 1971). Classic indirect laryngoscopy, for example, involving the insertion of a mirror into the pharynx and the protrusion of the tongue, prevents more than an artificial vowel sound being produced. The speed of vocal fold vibration produces only a blurred image of the superficial surface unless a stroboscopic light source is used. Little or nothing is seen of the vertical component of vocal fold vibration. High speed photography and endoscopy are equally disconcerting for the speaker.

Electrolaryngography is a non-invasive technique based on the monitoring of the varying electrical impedance of the vibrating vocal folds by means of two gold-plated guard ring electrodes superficially applied to the skin of the neck on each wing of the thyroid cartilage. The notion of electrical impedance monitoring which is basic to the design of the electrolaryngograph was introduced by Fabre (1957) in his 'glottograph', but its implementation in the present device is quite different. These differences, the operation of the electrolaryngograph, and its output waveform, Lx, have been described in detail in Fourcin and Abberton (1971), and Fourcin (1974, 1982). Here, it is sufficient to emphasise that Lx provides information about the closed phase of the vocal fold vibratory cycle. High-speed photography (Fourcin,

1974) confirms that the waveform is positive-going for increasing vocal fold closure and each peak corresponds to maximum contact between the folds; the leading edge of the waveform gives a precise indication of the beginning of the closure phase because closure normally occurs much more rapidly than opening. The Lx waveform does not give explicit information about glottal aperture size and, for this reason, is called a laryngograph rather than a glottograph. (A true glottograph gives information about the glottis which is the volume between the vocal folds). The term electrolaryngography is often used to distinguish the monitoring technique it makes possible from the radiographic method of enhancing soft laryngeal tissue which is known as laryngography (Landman, 1970).

Lx Waveforms

Vocal fold vibration is a complex three-dimensional motion. The horizontal opening and closing movements of the vocal folds to and from the midline are familiar from views in the laryngoscope mirror and introductory textbook illustrations, but the less well described vertical component of the vibratory cycle is extremely important in the effective production of voice. Just prior to phonation the vocal folds are approximated by the rotation of the arytenoid cartilages, and as the pulmonic egressive airstream passing up the trachea flows it increases in velocity and sucks the vocal folds together, very rapidly, from the bottom upwards — an example of the Bernoulli effect. The folds then peel apart more slowly, again from the bottom upwards (as subglottal air pressure builds up), and air flows into the vocal tract. In the normal voice this cycle is repeated with great regularity, over a range of frequencies dependent on the length and tension of the speaker's vocal folds: an adult man may have a fundamental frequency range of about 80 Hz to 200 Hz, and an adult woman a range from 140 Hz to 310 Hz, in conversational speech. In citation forms, expressive reading or excitement this range is extended. For the greater part of these ranges the speaker will use 'normal' or 'modal' voice, or vocal register. At the top end of his range a speaker may, on occasion, use the falsetto register, produced with thin, stretched vocal folds with a much-reduced vertical component in the vibration. At the lowest part of his range a speaker will typically have the creaky register available. This type of voice is produced with thick, slack folds and a low air-flow rate. Figure 4.1 shows speech and Lx waveforms for these three phonation types or registers. In normal or 'chest' voice the rapid closing phase produced by the Bernoulli effect is clearly different from the slower opening

Figure 4.1: Speech and Lx Waveforms from an Adult Female Speaker for a Sustained [a]

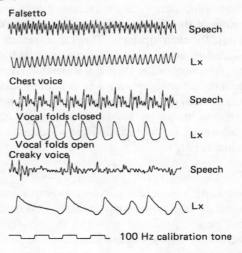

phase of the vibratory cycle as the folds peel apart. In falsetto, opening and closing rates are more nearly equal and the waveform more like that of a simple, sinusoidal, vibration. In creaky voice, closure is rapid but opening extremely slow; cycles of alternating large and small duration and amplitude also occur. Each of these three types of vibration may be accompanied by audible friction or breathiness, produced either by a longer open phase for each cycle or by incomplete antero-posterior closure of the vocal folds. In the former case, closing and opening rates will be more nearly equal.

Fundamental Frequency Monitoring and the Voiscope®

The rate of vibration of the vocal folds is continually changing in normal speech. This fundamental frequency, Fx, variation is rule-governed and provides the major physical correlate of the prosodic and paralinguistic pitch systems of intonation. The electrolaryngograph, incorporated into a device called a Voiscope®, provides a maximally accurate way of monitoring and displaying these patterns in a non-transient manner on an oscilloscope screen. The visual display is of a trace rising and falling in sympathy with the pitch of the speaker's voice. These contours are displayed on a logarithmic (octave) scale to correspond to our perception of pitch so that the Fx contours for a high-pitched voice appear higher up the screen than those for a low voice but the pattern for each is the same. Since the derivation of Fx from Lx is accomplished in real time (unlike the microphone-based cepstral analysis, for example (Noll, 1967) where only an average value for each laryngeal period is computed) the display of fundamental frequency that is provided shows cycle by cycle variation as well as overall contour. Thus, gaps appear for voiceless segments, and normal, regular, vocal fold vibration produces a smooth trace with only small perturbations for voiced obstruent consonants. Creaky voice and other irregular types of vibration show a broken ragged trace (see Figure 4.2). Both Lx and Fx can be of great value in remedial work and the basis of their use is described below in the section on speech therapy.

Figure 4.2: Fundamental Frequency, Fx, Contours for the Utterance '(the) sun was stronger than *he* was' from a Normal Man's Laryngograph, Lx Waveform. Each step corresponds to one vocal fold vibration

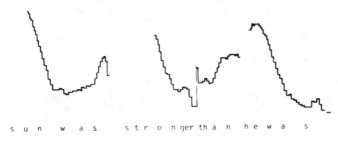

s u n   w a s   s t r o n ger tha n   he w a   s

Fx

Using the Lx waveform as the input makes it possible to show these contours without any averaging. In this way, small closure to closure variations can be clearly seen. For example: the breaks in the trace for the voiceless [st] in 'stronger' and the [h] in 'he'; the reduction in Fx for the [g] closure and the subsequent jump up for release; and the utterance-final irregularity due to creaky voice.

Quantitative Description of Vocal Fold Vibration Using Electrolaryngograph Recordings

The electrolaryngograph signal, Lx, can be recorded on an ordinary tape-recorder; stereo recordings are typically made, with speech on one channel and Lx on the other. (See Chapter 1 for further discussion on recording and storing speech.) Large amounts of data from spontaneous speech or reading can thus be collected and conveniently stored. Fundamental frequency information from a large sample of speech can be summarised, in a compact visual representation, by the use of a statistical analysis of the probability distribution of larynx periods. The resulting fundamental frequency range distributions (see Figure 4.3) correspond well with our auditory impression of wide or narrow pitch ranges, and the clearly visible modes or peaks (corresponding to a speaker's preferred fundamental frequency) correspond with our perception of high and low voices (Abberton, 1976; Fourcin and Abberton, 1976).

Figure 4.3: Microcomputer Based Measures of Voice Range and Regularity.

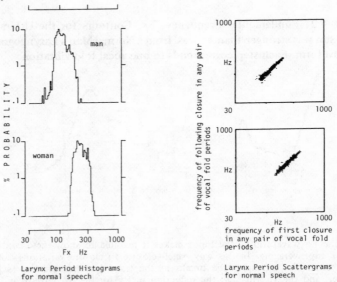

Larynx Period Histograms
for normal speech

Larynx Period Scattergrams
for normal speech

Just as larynx frequency contours can be easily derived from closure period measurements in the laryngograph waveform, so also can long-term histogram plots be obtained.

The two examples on the left show the probabilities of different larynx frequencies in terms of the number of occurrences of different length periods when two normal speakers read a standard text. The logarithmic frequency range from 10Hz to 1KHz has been divided into 100 equal bins and the height of the histogram at a bin position shows the relative number of vocal fold closures.

The two examples on the right indicate the scatter between adjacent periods in the same speech samples. A very regular voice activity is then associated with a well-defined diagonal distribution. Creaky voice in the male speech is associated with a widening of the distribution at the low frequency end in the scattergram — as well as perturbation of the histogram.

The standard text takes approximately two minutes to read.

Electrolaryngography in Speech Pathology

It has always been the aim of the electrolaryngography work originating from University College London to provide basic information not only on normal phonatory processes and fundamental frequency patterning but also on a range of laryngeal disorders, and, furthermore, to develop associated practical methods of vocal therapy for the reduction of these disorders. Fourcin (1982) points out that (i) in the assessment of vocal pathology it is essential to produce evaluations which relate to voice production, and that (ii) the electrolaryngograph is well suited to this purpose since its output is directly related to the events in the cycle of vocal fold vibration (the closing and closed phases) which are most important to the production of speech sounds: the vocal tract receives maximum excitation when it is isolated from the sub-glottal cavities by the closed vocal folds. Disorders of phonation will most likely be associated with the closing and closed phases of vocal fold vibration.

Abnormal Lx

A voice with an abnormal excitation may be characterised physically by irregular or otherwise imperfect vocal fold vibration throughout an utterance, or by only short sections of abnormal or inadequate vibration which nevertheless auditorily colour the speech continually. These points of inadequacy typically occur at major pitch changes (nuclear tones) or in association with certain oral articulations such as the lingua-laryngeal adjustments needed for velar consonants. In both these cases the aerodynamics of laryngeal airflow are disturbed and the speaker cannot produce symmetrical vocal fold vibration.

Normal vocal folds are of equal mass and stiffness and their mucus covering provides consistent viscosity. These physical parameters may be disturbed in a variety of pathological conditions: mass can be increased on one fold by a growth such as a polyp or a carcinoma; stiffness asymmetry results from unilateral paralysis; and viscosity is altered in infections such as laryngitis, or when the folds are abnormally dry for other reasons. Figure 4.4 shows the effect on Lx waveforms of pathological conditions.

Abnormal Lx waveforms have been presented and discussed in a number of studies. The first such study (Fourcin and Abberton, 1971) illustrated typical waveforms from speakers with unilateral vocal fold paralysis, ventricular vibration, and laryngitis, and the observation was made, for the first time, that phonation is not necessarily con-

Figure 4.4: Abnormal Waveforms.

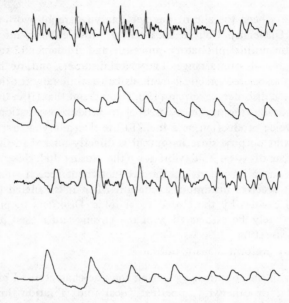

Two pairs of waveforms are shown. In each case the upper trace is a speech pressure waveform and the lower waveform shows the corresponding vocal fold closure information derived from a laryngograph: the Lx waveform. In each case the utterance 'stronger' was used and the activity relates to vowel onset.

The top pair were obtained from a patient with laryngitis. The Lx waveform is very irregular from period to period. The shape of each closure peak differs from its neighbour, and the normally sharp vertical movement to closure is sometimes quite gradual – and is then associated with a correspondingly smaller speech pressure peak. In addition, closure period regularity is variable – the space between successive Lx peaks is erratic.

The lower pair of traces were obtained from a patient with a uni-lateral paralysis. Here only one vocal fold is controlled normally by the speaker. As the speaker attempts to change his Fx contour considerable irregularity of both degree of closure – as shown by the heights of the Lx waveform peaks – and period occur. The shapes of individual closures are not markedly abnormal, however, since the contacting fold surfaces are not themselves impaired.

Vocal fold closure positive going. 0.5 s duration for each sample.

sistently and uniformly impaired in a pathological condition, and that a failure found repeatedly in one part of a particular intonation pattern may not be found elsewhere. Fourcin and Abberton (1976) show Lx waveforms with the corresponding pressure-time speech waveforms from speakers with unilateral paralysis, a pedunculate polyp (pre- and post-operatively) and from a normal speaker who had had an intramuscular injection of atropine to produce artificially dry vocal folds. In all the pairs of waveforms the simplicity of the Lx waveform compared with the complexity of the acoustic waveform allows the nature of the physical impairment of vocal fold vibration to be seen and interpreted in physical terms (Fourcin and Abberton, 1976: p. 118). Wechsler (1976a, b; 1977) studied vocal fold vibration before, during and after treatment for twenty subjects with inflammatory conditions or disorders of muscular control. Voice quality was assessed with the help of standard qualitative laryngologists' and speech therapists' judgments and patients' opinions, and of Lx waveforms.

Fourcin (1982) interprets normal Lx waveform shapes in terms of the five features listed below and points out that in pathology the Lx waveform can usefully be interpreted with reference to these five features to derive an indication of the nature and degree of the disorder.

(a) Uniform Lx peaks are likely to be associated with a correspondingly uniform acoustic output.
(b) Sharply defined Lx contact implies good acoustic excitation of the vocal tract.
(c) Long closure duration (contact plus separation) is likely to be associated with well-defined relatively undamped formants.
(d) Regular sharply defined contact periodicity will give a well-defined pitch.
(e) Progressive change in sharply defined Lx period lengths will be associated with a smoothly changing voice pitch.

In summary it is important to realise that there is no unique relationship between a pathological Lx waveform and a given anatomical or physiological condition. A *physical* interpretation of the waveform in terms of mass, tension, symmetry and conductivity is possible and this understanding supplements, but does not replace, standard visual examination by laryngoscopy.

Abnormalities of Fundamental Frequency

It is important from a theoretical point of view as well as from a clinical standpoint to realise that the laryngeal (and, incidentally, supra-glottal) components of a perceived voice quality do not depend only on consistent or long-term 'settings' of the speech apparatus. The dynamic features associated with changing fundamental frequency interact with variations in phonation type and play an essential role in giving the characteristic auditory colour to a voice. The following fundamental frequency characteristics may be impaired: (a) smoothness of Fx contour; (b) Fx contour shape; (c) Fx range; and (d) distribution of frequencies within the overall Fx range.

The derivation of Fx from Lx is accomplished in real time and on a cycle by cycle basis with no averaging. Thus every detail of the timing of successive vocal fold closures can be examined. Fourcin and Abberton (1971) and Abberton and Fourcin (1978) show typical Fx contours for English intonation patterns from a normal speaker: the Fx traces are smooth, reflecting regular vocal fold vibration, and show clearly defined changes associated with the words of greatest semantic importance in the utterances. The only departures from smooth contours are, as described above, gaps in the Fx traces for voiceless segments, and a broken trace for the normal brief use of creaky voice at low fundamental frequencies. In Fx contours from speakers with larynx problems, on the other hand, the regularity may be disturbed in predictable ways. In cases of extreme mechanical abnormality regular symmetrical vibration is impossible, broken traces are produced throughout, and no clear perception of pitch changes is produced. Often, however, vibration may become irregular or cease altogether only at certain points, particularly at major pitch changes. When a voiced obstruent consonant is produced the normal momentary lowering of fundamental frequency may be replaced by a cessation of voicing. Although stretches of Fx remain regular the disturbed portions are sufficient to give an impression of continuous abnormality, because of our auditory sensitivity to random variation in the timing characteristics of vocal fold vibration. Fourcin (1982) gives Fx traces for an utterance including a high falling nuclear tone and a voiced velar plosive from the same speaker (a) with normal vocal folds, and (b) when his vocal folds are abnormally dry following an intramuscular injection of atropine. The disturbances described above as well as the stretches of regular vibration are clearly seen.

A great deal of electrolaryngograph work has been carried out on the description, measurement and remediation of abnormal fundamental frequency in hearing-impaired speakers. The original work (with adults) and the relevant fundamental frequency and linguistic parameters are described and illustrated in Fourcin and Abberton (1971) and Abberton and Fourcin (1975). Because of lack of adequate auditory monitoring deaf speakers are likely to have abnormal voices with defects in all the four areas of Fx patterning listed above. Regularity of vibration and Fx contour shape are typically two major areas of difficulty; phonation may be in falsetto or creaky registers (inter-mittently or continuously) and contrastive use of pitch changes lacking or rudimentary. (See Fourcin and Abberton, 1971; Abberton and Fourcin, 1972, 1975 and Abberton *et al.*, 1977, for illustrations.) Wirz and Anthony (1979) show Fx traces for deaf children illustrating improvement in vocal fold regularity through Voiscope® training and also improvements in overall Fx level and the beginnings of intonation control — all features which had previously been moni-tored and improved in adults as described in the publications referred to above. King and Parker (1980) similarly describe the use of electro-laryngograph techniques when considering the importance of prosodic features in speech work with deaf children.

Both regularity of vocal fold vibration and the use of the contrastive pitch and rhythm patterns of intonation contribute importantly to perceived normal and abnormal voice quality and are essential para-meters to consider in clinical assessment. Both can be examined and described using electrolaryngograph techniques with oscilloscope displays or hard copy. (Interactive techniques with Lx and Fx visual displays are highly effective in changing perception and production of vibration type and fundamental frequency patterning; they are des-cribed below.)

Fundamental frequency range, and distribution of frequencies within that range, are also important indices of vocal performance, and they are capable of compact quantitative expression using Fx histo-grams suitable for inclusion in case notes. The effects of pathology can be clearly seen. In a normal speaker the Fx probability distribution is clearly defined with prominent modes (Abberton, 1976; Fourcin, 1982). The loss of the high or low ends of a speaker's range with, for example, inadequate vocal fold lubrication and viscosity are easily visible (Fourcin, 1982), as are the extension of the low frequency end of the distribution and lack of peaks seen, for example, with prolonged smoking (Abberton, 1976). The effects of surgery and therapy can be clearly indicated in this way: Fourcin (1982) and Abberton *et al.* (1977) show the extension of Fx range produced in deaf adults after work with an interactive Fx display. Similarly, Fourcin and Abberton (1976) and Wechsler (1977) show histograms for patients before and after treatment of laryngeal disorders, either by surgery or speech therapy. The Lx waveform provides an excellent basis for this sort of analysis since the beginning of each closure is indicated with a greater precision than is at present possible with other methods of analysis, and the simple form of the Lx waveform lends itself to real time analysis in which a simple algorithm identifies the start of onset for each vocal fold closure (Fourcin and Abberton, 1976; Fourcin, 1982). Figure 4.5 illustrates Fx histograms for speakers with disorders of laryngeal control.

Figure 4.5: Larynx Period Histograms for Abnormal Speech.

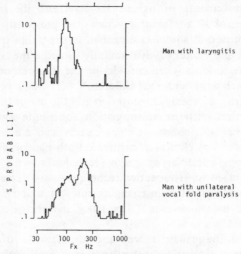

The normal larynx frequency histogram, plotted in this way, has a well-defined frequency range and shows a small number of dominant modes. Any pathology tends to show some deviation from these simple features. Laryngitis is often associated with frequency irregularity and restricted range around the main mode. Unilateral paralysis is also typically related to frequency irregularity but covers a much larger frequency range. These analyses are based on the same standard text as for Figure 4.3.

Clinical Applications of Electrolaryngography

The previous sections have shown how the electrolaryngograph can contribute to our knowledge of the definition of vocal pathology and its perceptual effects. The laryngograph work has always been explicitly oriented towards clinical therapeutic applications as well as theoretical in the study of pathological speech production and perception. Although, therefore, it is rather artificial to describe the work under separate Pathology and Clinical headings, since the techniques and findings we have described are now quite widely employed, abroad as well as in the UK, it is worth commenting on the main current clinical applications of electrolaryngography.

The earliest clinical work using interactive visual feedback techniques with a dynamic display of fundamental frequency (Voiscope®) was with profoundly deaf adults. It is clear that with phonetically and linguistically informed guidance these speakers can benefit from the visual information derived directly from their vocal folds to learn new patterns of laryngeal control and to monitor their speech in new ways. Subsequent studies showed that young children and adolescents can also benefit from the technique. Fourcin (1980) describes some results obtained with children showing how their perception of a basic intonation contrast improved as a result of linguistically oriented production work using the Voiscope®. The enhancement of perception as well as production is essential for the maintenance of new speech skills no matter what pathology is involved.

Abnormal vocal fold vibration is a common problem with hearing impaired speakers and along with intonation patterning is a focus of attention in therapy with laryngograph techniques. Dysphonia in normally hearing speakers with laryngeal problems provides a range of conditions open to investigation, description and remediation using the laryngograph and Voiscope®. Once again, the clinical focus is on the interaction of perception and production in bringing about voice improvement as the speaker becomes aware of what he is doing and what he sounds like by having his attention drawn to dynamic visual displays.

The two most recent applications of the laryngograph and Voiscope® in assessment and remediation are in external electro-cochlear stimulation of people with acquired total deafness (Fourcin *et al.*, 1978; Rosen, Fourcin and Moore, 1981; Fourcin *et al.*, 1983), and combined with xeroradiographic imaging (Berry *et al.*, 1982a, b). In external electro-cochlear stimulation the laryngograph has been used as an essential research tool providing the acoustically totally deaf speaker with prosodic, paralinguistic and segmental voicing information to supplement lip-reading. The non-invasive microphone-based prosthesis that has resulted from this work and the signal processing facilities that it provides are the direct outcome of laryngograph work on matching the input signal to a patient's needs and new auditory receptive capabilities. Speech productive and receptive rehabilitation is enhanced, and progress monitored in qualitative and quantitative terms, by the methods described in this chapter.

Combined xeroradiography and electrolaryngography (X.E.L.) are providing qualitative visual information on dysfunction of the larynx and vocal tract, unavailable by other means, in terms both of clear anatomical images and Lx waveforms. Visual feedback methods are used in therapy, and progress monitored by this X.E.L. technique. Among others, patients with functional dysphonias and even laryngectomees are benefiting from the approach. X.E.L. technique is discussed further in Chapter 6.

Vocal Therapy Using Electrolaryngography

Dynamic displays of Lx and/or Fx on oscilloscope screens provide the basis for a highly effective method of therapy based on reinforcing or error-correcting visual feedback (Fourcin and Abberton, 1976). These displays are motivating for the speaker undergoing therapy and often produce improvements not possible with other techniques. The principle of using visual displays in speech therapy is essentially that of pattern matching: a model pattern is displayed on the screen (or sketched on a card) and the speaker compares his own output (on the screen) with the target. He thus receives correcting or reinforcing visual feedback. In this way both perception and production are improved by establishing auditory and kinaesthetic awareness of one's own vocal patterns. Observation of Lx is used to establish or change vocal fold vibration type or register and Fx for work on pitch height, timing, intonation, and regularity of vocal fold vibration. The factors that make for successful 'biofeedback' therapy of this kind are as follows.

1. The visual feedback provided, of both Lx and Fx, is patterned; the patient is not simply given binary Yes/No information about the correctness of his utterance. In other words he can see where and how he has gone wrong.

2. In the early stages of work with the laryngograph (Lx display) and Voiscope® (Fx display) the speaker receives immediate knowledge of results (KR). Any delay between speaking and seeing the traces would interfere with motor control. As therapy progresses, however, the speaker can have controlled delayed KR by turning the oscilloscope brilliance down, and only turning it up, to see the whole pattern he has produced, after he has made a judgment on its adequacy. This is clearly a most important stage in developing auditory and kinaesthetic awareness of new vocal habits, and in weaning the speaker away from the display. It is also a useful facility when the speaker is practising alone: with this type of therapy the therapist does not need to be present continuously.

3. It is important that the display of Fx is stored, not transitory, so that the whole pattern can be appreciated and studied. The ear

can process rapidly changing stimuli but for visual processing the whole pattern needs to be available at the same time. Continuous feedback during spontaneous speech can be obtained using the FLOW option: a continuous right to left flowing display is available which can be frozen at any particular moment so that a particular utterance can be examined.

4. A logarithmic (or octave) scale of fundamental frequency is used to conform to our auditory perception of pitch. As described above, this means that speakers with very different average fundamental frequencies will produce contours of the same shape, but higher or lower on the screen, corresponding in a natural and simple way to our normal experience of pitch patterns. Acoustic auditory targets are thus provided rather than articulatory instruction (Abberton, Ashby and Fourcin, 1976).

5. An important practical advantage when working in schools and clinics is that the laryngograph and Voiscope®, operating from surface electrodes, are impervious to ambient acoustic noise. Their displays are thus accurate and uncontaminated. With some speakers, however, a microphone input rather than one derived directly from the speaker's larynx is more convenient (e.g. with cerebral palsied subjects) and a microphone input is available as a Voiscope® option. Lx, of course, is not available from a microphone-based device.

6. The success of therapy using visual feedback depends on the use of accurate displays and on a graded programme of work using phonetic and linguistic knowledge of speech production, and of phonological patterning in the language concerned. As far as visual study of Lx is concerned this involves awareness of (1) the need for adequate acoustic excitation of the vocal tract (modal voice register) in order to produce acceptable vowels and consonants — not only supraglottal articulatory movements are important; and (2) knowledge of different phonation types. The Fx display clearly shows voiced-voiceless contrasts and the importance of duration differences to English rhythm and intelligibility (Fourcin and Abberton, 1971). Intonation control and improvement are achieved by the teaching of simple rules. For English, these include the correct, context-determined placement of the nuclear syllable (the most stressed syllable in a word group), and the choice of nuclear tone (rising, falling, falling-rising, rising-falling) to convey the required linguistic or non-verbal paralinguistic information (O'Connor and Arnold, 1973; Brazil, 1975). For

example, the statement 'This tea tastes good' has different meanings depending on which word receives the major stress, signalled in most cases by a falling nuclear tone. Rising or falling-rising tones would typically signal doubt or questioning, or simply continuity and lack of finality. Which word is treated as nuclear depends on what is considered new information, the focus of attention, in the light of what has been said before — 'good' not 'bad', 'tea' rather than 'coffee', for example.

The approach to teaching and learning, therefore, is essentially a cognitive one rather than an attempt to teach a repertoire of utterances as wholes through conditioning. Rather, the emphasis is on the learning of patterns and rules for their use together with the enhancement of self-monitoring.

Conclusion

We have tried to outline, in a simple way, a method of monitoring, assessing and measuring vocal fold vibration in speech, and the principles of a type of therapy that it makes possible. The approach is highly effective and often brings about improvements that were not possible with more traditional techniques. The principles and techniques we have described were developed at University College, London and are now also being used in schools and clinics in Britain and several other countries. One of the aims of the original work was to reduce the voice problems of hearing-impaired speakers (Fourcin and Abberton, 1971). This has continued and been developed in the cochlear stimulation work (Fourcin *et al.*, 1980). The approach is also used with a wide range of voice difficulties in normally hearing patients (Wechsler, 1977; Berry *et al.*, 1982a, b) and, in principle, is suitable for any speaker with problems of rhythm, pitch control and phonation. Many developmental, pathological and therapeutic studies remain to be done in the areas of voice quality and intonation, and the laryngograph provides the possibility of adding quantitative information to the investigator's qualitative evaluation.

5 AEROMETRY

James Anthony and Nigel Hewlett

Introduction

The view that speech is breathing changed in some way has been expressed by many phoneticians over the last century and has been accepted, of course, as obviously true. Passy (1914) perhaps expressed it most concisely; 'All speech sounds have their origin in a single physiological act – respiration – modified in various ways. We may therefore consider as being included in the organs of speech, firstly the respiratory system, and secondly the structures which may serve to modify respiration'. More recently, Fenn (1958) introduced an engineering viewpoint, 'Vocalisation has evolved as an ingenious exploitation of the breathing mechanism for the purpose of meaningful communication'.

There has, however, been a curious lack of interest in what the implications of these statements might be with regard to the production process of speech and little investigation into what 'modification' means. How is respiration changed to ensure a supply of air on demand to the speech mechanism? This kind of modification could be considered a change of organisation operating over the long term.

The interaction of the movements of the tongue, lips, soft-palate and larynx modifies the airstream from the lungs to form a modulated airflow from mouth and nose of which the audible part is the acoustic signal of speech. This is the short-term modification where voicing and articulation determine the instantaneous rate of flow through the vocal tract.

The basic requirement for sound production is a subglottal pressure raised above ambient and a volume of air within the lungs adequate for the utterance. These two quantities, the pressure difference across, and the flow of air through, the larynx, multiplied together have the physical dimension of power and as the product of power and time is energy, we have the means of quantifying the aerodynamic effort that the human being expends in speech.

The volume of air within the lungs is generally so much greater than the immediate requirements for speech that it could be said that air is supplied 'on demand'. The pressure below the larynx is then, in a sense, more important than the flow and in speech is adjusted and controlled very precisely indeed. The speaker can maintain an average pressure to produce speech which will be judged subjectively by the listener as having a particular loudness and he can increase it above the average at certain instants to place stress on selected syllables (Ladefoged and McKinney, 1963). By the adjustment of the muscles of the larynx he can control the oscillatory characteristics of the vocal cords and the frequency of vibration will have the perceived quality of pitch. The movements of the lips, tongue and the soft-palate vary the dimensions of the cavity systems of nose and mouth, which modify the spectrum of the larynx source. The resulting output from the nose and the mouth is therefore an extremely complex acoustic signal.

Airflow measurement is essential to an understanding of how the short-term and the long-term modifications to the respiratory function interact and are synchronised. Only with detailed quantitative records can we study the response of the respiratory system to different speech tasks and begin to define normal and abnormal performance. For example, a disability in speaking which appears to be due to abnormal laryngeal function may, in fact, have its cause in the failure of the respiratory mechanism to provide adequate aerodynamic support for the phonatory and articulatory system.

Pathologies associated with the first (long-term) modification of breathing are primarily those in which the respiratory centre is affected. Parkinson's disease would be one example where laryngeal and thoracic problems lead to inefficient ventilation for speech. As another example, the reduced range of intonation and volume in the speech of many patients who have suffered a cerebrovascular accident may be ascribed to the reduced power of the lungs to provide suitable subglottal pressures throughout speech.

The most striking example of pathology associated with the second (short-term) modification must be that of the cleft-palate patient whose ability to apportion airflow through nose and mouth is severely reduced. However, any disability which decreases the efficiency of the valve action of the organs of the laryngeal and supra-laryngeal vocal tract must affect the speaker's ability to achieve the short-term changes in airflow that are required for speech.

This chapter is mainly concerned with the short-term analysis of speech airflow but it is often difficult to distinguish short-term and long-term in practice. Methods of measurement will first be discussed and the characteristics of normal articulatory waveforms will be described before considering clinical applications and typical results.

Measurement

To Menzies (1790) should probably go the honour of being the first to measure, or at least the first to describe the means of measuring, respiratory volumes and energy expenditure. This was simply a barrel, large enough to hold an adult, which had a close-fitting airtight collar at the neck to leave the head free (Figure 5.1). As the subject breathes his body volumes will increase and decrease, the airflow in and out of the barrel will vary accordingly and a spirometer connected by a pipe will then indicate how lung volume has changed. This technique, *plethysmography*, has been used ever since, though, of course, it has been developed in many ways (Haldane and Priestly, 1905; Draper, Ladefoged and Whitteridge, 1960; Bouhuys, Proctor and Mead, 1966). The main advantage of this system for respiratory and speech studies is that there is no restrictive mask on the face and no distortion of the acoustic signal; the main problem, however, is the difficulty of using the method routinely in the clinical speech assessment of adults

Figure 5.1:

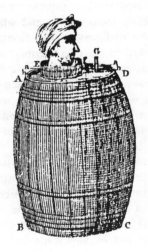

Source: From Menzies (1790)

and children. Modern plethysmographs have easy access and egress but there is still an inherent danger which is not acceptable. The other problems are the large volumes of air involved which seriously limit the frequency response and the need to provide air conditioning for the container to maintain constant temperature.

In the study of the aerodynamics of speech production simultaneous measurements are required, long-term of ventilation and short-term of articulation. Moreover, to investigate the flow waveforms of speech sounds separate measurements must be obtained from nose and mouth (Hewlett and Anthony, 1982). The plethysmograph approach is therefore unsuitable and the most appropriate method at the present time appears to be *pneumotachography*.

The principle of the pneumotach can perhaps be best explained by considering what happens when an airpressure is applied to the end of a tube, say, for example, by someone blowing, and the other end is open to the atmosphere. Obviously, air will pass down and out of the tube from the higher pressure to the lower and if conditions were reversed and the person sucked then a negative pressure (less than atmosphere) would be applied and air would be drawn up through the tube, through the mouth and into the lungs. Note that pressures are referred and measured with respect to atmospheric because the volume of atmospheric air being so vast we can consider its pressure constant.

In our tube the pressure applied is 'dropped' along its length and if it is a straight tube, all of the same material, then we can expect that the pressure difference will decrease linearly from end to end which means that the flow resistance is distributed linearly, also, along it. If now a concentrated resistance ('lumped' in electrical terms) were introduced midway along the tube, such as a constriction or a fine mesh screen, then, everything else being equal, the flow would be reduced and part of the applied pressure would exist across the resistance. Further, if the resistance were made very large (compared to that of the tube) then the pressure drop of the tube itself could be neglected.

The pneumotachographic head (flowhead for short) is a deceptively simple device but its design has been improved since its invention (Fleisch, 1925) to give good linearity between the pressure difference across the resistance (in modern types a fine wire gauze) and the volume velocity of the air through it. If the construction is symmetrical then, of course, the device is bi-directional and, because it has no moving parts, flow is proportional to pressure down to zero pressure and flow. Electronic transducers attached to the flowhead, and their amplifiers, give an output voltage proportional to pressure difference, with a good frequency response.

The flowhead is fitted into an anaesthetic mask which has a soft surround and is held firmly against the face by means of a head harness. The subject's head movements are not restricted and he can take up whatever sitting posture is most comfortable. There are three principal disadvantages, however, in the pneumotachograph method. First, there is the problem of air leakage at the mask edges, especially of expiratory speech air around the bridge of the nose, along the cheeks, under the chin and, where a divided mask with two flowheads is used, between mouth cavity and nose cavity. There is a need, clearly, for a new design of facemask for airflow recording, especially for children.

Second, though not a serious disadvantage in practice, is the fact that the flow resistance of the flowhead, which must be used, is not as low as it should be. The air to be measured passes through the measuring instrument and therefore its resistance should be smaller than that of the system being measured; it should not be high enough to impede respiration or hinder speech production but the lower the resistance the more gain is required in the amplifying system. In this study the Type F2 (19mm bore) manufactured by Mercury Electronics (Scotland) Ltd has been used. The expiratory resistance of the respiratory system can be taken to be between 2 and 5 ohms (1 ohm = $\frac{1 \text{cm aqua}}{1 \text{ litre/s}}$) (Rothenberg, 1968) and the resistance of the vocal tract (in series with the respiratory resistance) will vary from say, 0.5 ohm for open vowels to 100 ohms or more for fricatives. The resistance of the F2 head is of the same order having a nominal resistance of one ohm. This is not to say that the resistance is so high that it affects speech production; it is not noticeable to the normal speaker during speaking or breathing.

Third, the acoustic quality of the speech is affected adversely by the enclosure of the mouth and nose in the cavity of the mask. The effect is, as expected, more evident with speech sounds which have their acoustic energy concentrated at higher frequencies so that fricatives and sibilants tend to be lost but the quality is still quite adequate for the purpose of making a broad phonetic transcription. One, admittedly unsatisfactory, way round this problem is to make a separate tape-recording first without mask before airflow assessment and this is standard practice. Another, under investigation, is to record the speech from a microphone inside the mask.

Connected to each flowhead, nasal and oral, is a pressure transducer which gives a voltage change output proportional to the pressure difference change across the gauze; this is, as described earlier, proportional to the volume velocity (flow) through the pneumotach head. The ever changing waveform of speech airflow requires dynamic measurement and so the voltage output of the electronic amplifier for each transducer is applied to the amplifier of a high-speed ink-jet oscillograph which gives a change in position of a line, a trace, proportional to the voltage applied. We can see that first we measure flow in terms of pressure (aerodynamic), then pressure in terms of voltage (electrical) and then voltage in terms of movement (mechanical). Given that the relationship between each is known then the deflection of the trace can be calibrated in terms of flow. For example let us say that when there is a pressure difference of 1 cm Aq. (1 cm of water pressure) across the outlet pipes of the flowhead there is a flow of 42 l/min (42 litres per minute), that is, 700 ml/s (700 millilitres per second). This pressure applied to the transducer and its amplifier is arranged (normally) to give an output change of 1 volt which, when applied to the oscillograph amplifier, is arranged to give a deflection (normally) of 2 cm.

Then:-

Oral flow: 700 ml/s/1 cm Aq./1V/2 cm

or   340 ml/s/cm

To give a nasal trace comparable in overall size to that of the oral trace, it is necessary, for normal speech, to increase the gain of the oscillographic amplifier by four times, i.e. 1 volt will give a deflection of 8 cm.

Then:-

Nasal flow: 700 ml/s/1 cm Aq./1V/8 cm

or   85 ml/s/cm

Expiratory flow (outgoing from the lungs) results from positive pressures (above ambient) within the lungs. In contrast to general practice in respiratory measurement this is recorded as a deflection upwards on the oscillographic record because almost all speech is produced on egressive flow.

The amount of other data that can be displayed, for instance on a direct-writing ink-jet oscillograph such as the Mingograph, is limited, of course, only by the number of channels available. It is of great advantage in analysis to have other simultaneous measurements, for example, timing calibration, air volumes (by resetting integrators), laryngographic voicing waveforms (Fourcin, 1974; Anthony, 1978), the fundamental frequency of voicing (the 'pitch') and the speech acoustic waveform from an external microphone.

Figure 5.2: Experimental Arrangement for Recording the Airflow, Vocal Cord Vibration Waveform and the Acoustic Signal of Speech

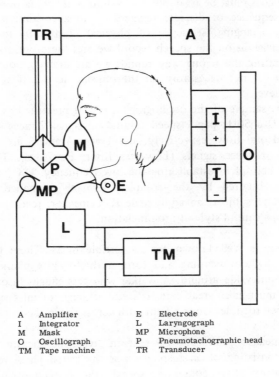

A	Amplifier	E	Electrode
I	Integrator	L	Laryngograph
M	Mask	MP	Microphone
O	Oscillograph	P	Pneumotachographic head
TM	Tape machine	TR	Transducer

Figure 5.2 shows the experimental arrangement for recording nasal and oral flow combined; for most speech investigations a divided mask is used and two separate sets of transducers and amplifiers are employed.

An Airflow Record of Normal Speech

An oscillographic record with all these kinds of data contains a wealth of information but the problems of analysis are eased considerably by breaking down the continuous stream of speech into manageable, smaller phonetic units. On intuitive grounds the speech signal is conceived, usually, as being the realisation of a sequence of discrete segments which may be represented as such at some higher level of neural encoding. Segmental divisions are not an intrinsic property of the physical speech output at the aerodynamic or acoustic level but the ultimate goal must be to develop a system of mapping rules which will map a sequence of discrete segments onto a continuous, and continuously changing, sequence of physical events. By imposing segmental divisions on the speech record we are, therefore, strictly speaking, operating the wrong way round; we are drawing boundaries that exist not (or not necessarily) at the physical level but at some more abstract level.

On the sample of the oscillographic record presented as Figure 5.3, Trace 2 is a 50Hz paper speed calibration signal. Traces 4 and 7 are nasal and oral flow respectively, and Traces 3 and 6 are the filtered versions of these signals (Low-pass filter, Fc=70Hz). This filtered signal is helpful in establishing the low frequency 'D.C.' flow which is often obscured by the complex formant resonances in voiced sounds. The subject, an adult male R.P. speaker, read the following passage in a careful style of pronunciation.

> Exmoor is well known for its terrible mists. These mists come down without warning and form a thick white blanket over all the countryside around. A walker who gets caught in one of these mists must take great care. It's easy enough to miss signposts on the open road, let alone a faint path across the moors.

The speaker produced the text in five 'Speech Breath Cycles', a cycle consisting of an inspiration as the initial phase followed by an expiratory phase containing speech (the 'Speech Breath Group'); the expiratory phase may, of course, contain one or more Speech Breath Groups.

Table 5.1 gives the figures for the volumes of oral and nasal air used in each of the breath groups in these data and the ratios.

A noticeable feature of the airflow record is that it indicates negative flows, both oral and nasal, at several points during actual speech

Figure 5.3: Channels 2-9 of the Airflow-voicing Record of the First Two Words of the Text: 'Exmoor is . . .'.

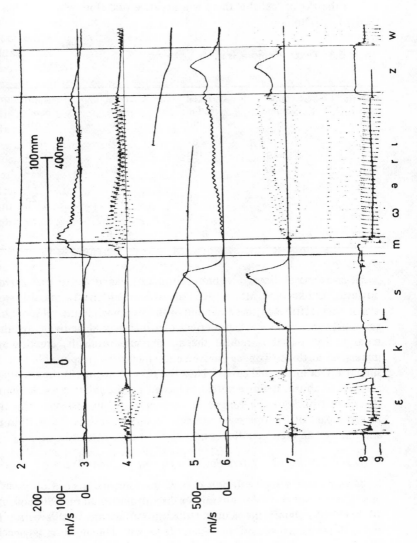

(i.e. as opposed to inspirations between breath groups). For example, during the /k/ of 'caught' there is a negative oral flow which reaches a peak of −102ml/s.

Table 5.1: Text: 'Exmoor is . . .'

Speech breath group	Oral volume (ml)	Nasal volume (ml)	Total nasal + oral	Ratio nasal to oral
1	374	61	435	0.16
2	449	153	602	0.34
3	425	78	503	0.18
4	262	85	347	0.32
5	262	65	327	0.25
Totals	1172	442	2214	—
Means	354.4	88.4	442.8	0.38

Negative nasal flows are more common than negative oral flows, however. Lubker and Moll (1965) also observed negative nasal flows, which they attributed to a lowering of the velum while the velopharyngeal port remained closed, the effect of which would be to enlarge the nasal cavity and thus reduce the air pressure inside it, creating an ingressive airflow. Tongue movements might be responsible for a similar effect in the oral cavity. Thus the /k/ of 'caught', in the example mentioned above, is immediately preceded by the /s/ of 'gets'. Perhaps the pulling back of the tongue at the release of the /s/ enlarged the forward part of the oral cavity which decreased the pressure within it and induced an ingressive flow of air.

Flow and Voicing Characteristics of Different Segment Types

In carrying out a segmentation of any instrumental record of speech one is, wherever possible, looking for discontinuities to indicate boundaries. Certain significant acoustic discontinuities are not revealed in an airflow-voicing record however. Thus for sequences of adjacent vowels, or vowels and voiced approximants, no attempt was made to draw in segment boundaries; acoustic spectral analysis of the waveform may help to suggest segment boundaries in such sequences. It is also worth emphasising that this type of record gives no information about place of articulation. So no segment boundary can be drawn within the /tk/ sequence in 'great care' for example, in which the /t/ was not released.

Figure 5.4: Nasal, Oral and Laryngographic Traces for a Selection of Oral Stops

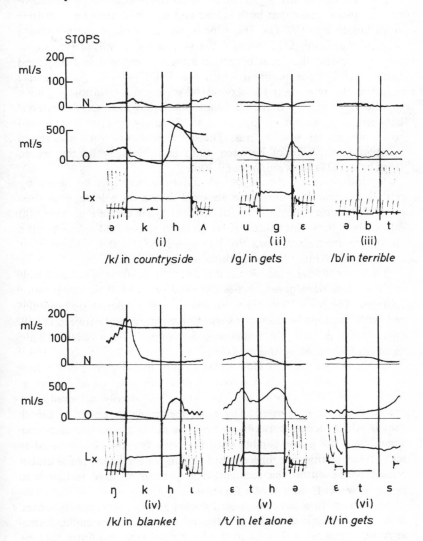

Oral Stops

Figure 5.4 shows examples from the record of voiced and voiceless stops occurring in several different phonetic environments. Only the N_f, O_f, and L_x traces are shown.

All the initial stops show a period of complete oral closure, which is released before the onset of vocal cord vibration. It is character-istic of this speaker that both voiced and voiceless stops have positive voice onset times (VOTs). This type of record provides a very accurate way of measuring VOT because the two factors involved (release of the closure and the onset of vibration) are monitored and displayed independently. The point at which the oral flow trace goes positive indicates the release, and the onset of vocal cord vibration is shown on the L_x trace. It is then a simple matter to measure the interval between them, and at a paper speed of 250 mm/s the error is estimated to be no greater than ± 2ms. The initial voiceless stops of stressed syllables have VOTs of between 40ms and 70ms, while the voiced stops have VOTs between 5ms and 30ms.

An indication of the degree of aspiration may also be gained by noting the peak oral flow rate achieved during the release. Peak flow rates for voiceless initial stops of stressed syllables were all over 500 ml/s, while those for voiced stops were all under 300 ml/s. But the /t/ of the unstressed word 'to' has values (VOT=20ms and peak air flow rate = 240 ml/s) similar to those for voiced stops.

There are several examples in the data of medial stops during which the oral flow trace never reaches the baseline, i.e. full closure is never achieved. The /b/ of 'terrible' is an example of a voiced stop pronoun-ced with incomplete closure. (Voiced stops occurring between sonor-ants, like this one, are sometimes pronounced with full-amplitude vocal cord vibration by this speaker.)

It is common to find incomplete closure in voiceless stops before /s/. The voiceless stops in 'Exmoor', 'mists' and 'gets' are all examples. Alternatively, oral closure may be only momentarily achieved, just before the stop is released. The most spectacular example of this is the /t/ which occurs between two vowels in the phrase 'let alone', in which the flow is comparable with that of a fricative. But it is inter-esting that in this case one can still distinguish a 'stop' phase and a release phase within the segment. The pattern of flow is therefore rather different from that of a fricative.

Some nasal flow may be present during an oral stop, usually where it follows a nasal. The /k/ of 'blanket' provides an example. But if anything but a small flow is involved the nasal trace can invariably be

observed to start descending steeply towards the baseline at the onset
of the oral stop.

**Figure 5.5: Nasal, Oral and Laryngographic Traces for a Selection of
Fricatives**

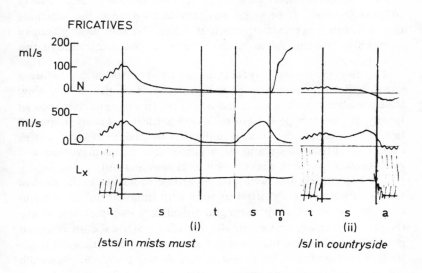

/sts/ in *mists must*   /s/ in *countryside*

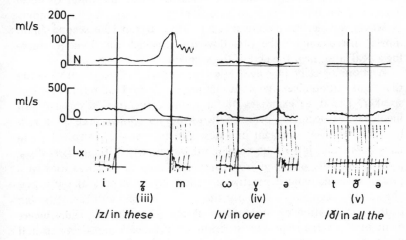

/z/ in *these*   /v/ in *over*   /ð/ in *all the*

Fricatives

Figure 5.5 shows the N_f, O_f, and the L_x traces for a selection of fricatives.

Fricatives undoubtedly involve greater air flow rates than any other segment type, and certain characteristic patterns of flow (characteristic at least of this speaker) emerge from the data.

In a vowel-fricative sequence oral flow generally rises steadily towards the end of the vowel and reaches its peak at the beginning of the fricative segment, throughout which the flow then gradually diminishes. The first /s/ in 'mists' provides a good illustration of this pattern.

The few examples of syllable initial fricatives occurring before a vowel indicate an opposite pattern, i.e. a gradual rise in oral flow which reaches a peak towards the end of the fricative and then reduces rapidly at the start of the vowel. Where a fricative occurs intervocalically, for example the /s/ in 'countryside' and the /θ/ in 'path across', the flow pattern appears to be a composite of the prevocalic and post-vocalic types, with peaks at both beginning and end.

The explanation for these oral flow trajectories lies in the relative timing between onset or offset of vocal cord vibration and the achievement of the required supralaryngeal articulatory configuration. Where the fricative occurs post-vocalically the offset of vocal cord vibration probably occurs a few milliseconds before the full constriction for the fricative segment has been achieved; and conversely, in prevocalic position the constriction may be released before the onset of vocal cord vibration.

Where a voiceless fricative occurs after a stop (the second /s/ in 'mists', for example) the oral flow rises through the fricative reaching a peak at or near the end of the segment.

A phonologically [+ voice] fricative, i.e. /z/, /v/ etc., is more often than not pronounced without actual vocal cord vibration by this speaker. The three examples of fully voiced fricatives in the data (all involving /ð/ occurring between two sonorant segments) reveal a very low and relatively constant oral flow. Of the rest (i.e. [+ voice] fricatives pronounced without vocal cord vibration), different oral flow patterns may be observed from the ones found in voiceless fricatives. In a post-vocalic voiced fricative oral flow does not peak at the beginning of the segment, but nearer the end, indicating a different timing in the coordination of onset of vocal cord vibration and the achievement of the articulatory constriction. In prevocalic position the oral flow pattern is similar to that of voiceless fricatives.

One would probably expect lower oral flows in voiced, as opposed to voiceless, fricatives. However, segment type is by no means the only significant variable affecting the flow rate. The degree of stress with which the word is spoken is probably at least as important, and the flow rates of voiced and voiceless fricatives in the data certainly show considerable overlapping. Similar remarks could be made concerning duration, although the voiced fricatives in these data are generally shorter than the voiceless.

Where a fricative occurs after a nasalised vowel (as in 'mists', for example) some nasal flow usually persists into the fricative. However, on these occasions the nasal flow trace is descending sharply towards the baseline during the onset of the fricative.

Nasals

Figure 5.6 shows the N_f, O_f and L_x traces for a selection of nasal consonants.

Nasal flow occurs without exception during nasal consonants, reaching a peak of at least 65 ml/s. Typically, the nasal flow trace starts to rise from the baseline during the preceding segment and continues to rise throughout the nasal, reaching a peak at or near the end of the segment. The /n/ of 'enough' (see Figure 5.6) shows a typical nasal flow trajectory, associated with zero oral flow and voicing.

Most of the nasal stops in the data exhibit a full oral closure. However, there is moderate oral flow during the /m/ of 'form' and during the /n/ of 'signposts', which may indicate an incomplete closure in these cases.

The only examples of voiceless (or partially voiceless) nasals in the data occur after /s/. Nasal flows in these segments consequently tend to be large. Thus the /m/ of 'must', in 'mists must' is voiceless and has a peak nasal flow rate of 178 ml/s.

Vowels

Vowels are typically produced with a moderate, and relatively constant, rate of oral flow. But in a transition from vowel to voiceless consonant the periodic waveform of the unfiltered trace near the end of the vowel rears up from the baseline. This corresponds to a steep rise in the filtered trace. Good examples are the transition to /k/ of 'walker' and the transition to /s/ of 'miss'. It is as though the quasi-steady flow from the lungs is acting as a carrier for the periodic wave as vocal cord vibration tails off.

Figure 5.6: Nasal, Oral and Laryngographic Traces for a Selection of Nasal Stops

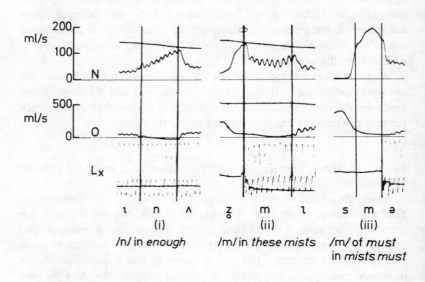

/n/ in *enough*   /m/ in *these mists*   /m/ of *must* in *mists must*

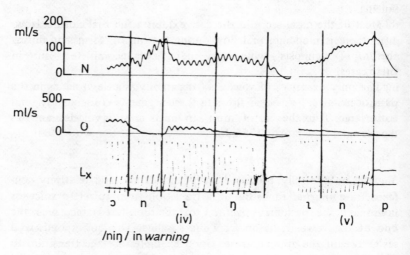

/niŋ/ in *warning*

The occurrence of nasal flow during vowels is by no means entirely predictable for this speaker. There is always some nasal flow where a vowel is adjacent to a nasal consonant, although the amount and duration varies considerably. Thus nasal flow reaches zero during the vowel which occurs between the two nasal stops in 'known', for example, whereas in the word 'warning' nasal flow rises steadily from about two-thirds of the way through the first vowel and continues throughout the word. Onset and offset of nasal flow is typically smooth and unhurried during a vowel sound.

There are also examples of nasal flow during a vowel which cannot be attributed to the presence of a nasal consonant. The most notable case in the present data is the vowel in 'path'. Although there is no nasal consonant in the vicinity, the nasal flow during this vowel reaches 125 ml/s, higher than that of any of the nasal consonants in the same breath group!

Applications in Speech Pathology and Therapeutics

This analysis of one type of normal speech gives an insight into the general characteristics of the speech airflow that results from phonation and articulation and patterns such as these provide sets of data with which to compare, dynamically and quantitatively, the waveform of pathological speech. In cleft-palate speech for example, we find that the shape of the trace for /s/ following a vowel is changed, the oral flow is less, the nasal flow is greater than the normal and the difference gives an indication of the goodness of closure at the nasal port; where /s/ follows a nasal we can check to see if the nasal flow falls to zero, as it should, before the fricative. In one type of stammering certain short-term changes occur with abnormal laryngeal function when syllables are repeated, while for other types the long-term organisation of lung volume usage shows how the ventilatory balance between the needs of respiration and the demands of speech production has been disturbed.

Quantitative airflow analysis is a new phonetic and clinical technique. When a body of information on the patterns of normal speech (especially of children between 3 and 5 years old) becomes available it will be possible to define precisely the *ways in which* and *the amounts by which* the patient deviates from the norm. As our knowledge increases the technique becomes more and more useful by illustrating clearly the phonetic consequences of abnormal production processes and by supplementing other methods of observation such as fibre-optic endoscopy and video-fluoroscopy. The greatest challenge, however, lies in establishing the relationships between the objective airflow record and the subjective judgement of intelligibility and voice quality.

Airflow measurement, by its very nature, should be able to shed light on many speech problems. Transducer development has been rapid (Anthony and MacLachlan, 1969) but there are still certain difficulties associated with segmentation and synchronisation of the airflow recording with other articulatory observation (fibre-optic endoscopy and X-ray) and with acoustic (spectrographic) data. As experience is gained it is clear that measurements of sub-glottal and supra-glottal pressure would greatly aid interpretation of the records, allow nasal and oral flow resistance to be calculated and begin to give an understanding of the pattern of energy cost, in speaking, to the human being. Airflow investigations using various techniques have been made into a number of communication disorders; there is, however, little routine clinical application of the results as yet. A number of these studies are considered here and examples of pathological speech records are given to stimulate further research.

The area of cleft-palate assessment is obviously one where aerometry should play a large part; as yet, however, the technique is not widely applied. For example, the proceedings of the 8th Conference of the British College of Speech Therapists contains four papers on cleft-palate and velopharyngeal incompetency, only one of which discusses aerometry. Nevertheless, the potential of the technique has been recognised and in the 1970 ASHA proceedings of the Workshop on Speech and the Dento-facial Complex, there is a section 'The State of the Art' which describes various assessment methods. Lubker (1970) considers that pneumotachography using a facemask is probably the most reliable. In Quigley *et al.* (1963, 1964) and Quigley (1967) the view is put forward that nasal airflow can act as an index of velopharyngeal competency. Other researchers, however, such as Lubker and Moll (1965), Warren and Ryon (1967) and Lubker and Schweiger (1969) warn that a number of other factors need to be taken into consideration.

Important aspects of nasality are discussed in Scully (1980). Both aerometry and spectrography (see Chapter 2 for a description of this technique) are used because it is felt that they can help build up a picture of the complex ways in which the two cavities (oral and nasal) are linked in speech production. It is also pointed out that perception tests will be needed to determine how acoustic features correlate with auditory judgements of speech therapists. The first step towards establishing the relationship between articulatory and acoustic descrip-

Figure 5.7: The Nasal and Oral Airflow of a Child with a Cleft Palate Whistling

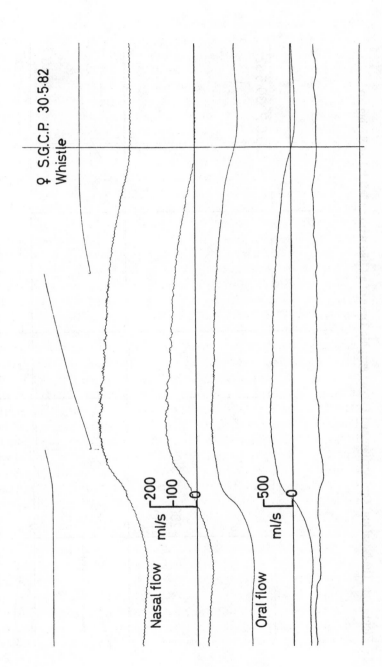

Figure 5.8: The Nasal and Oral Airflow and Laryngographic Trace of a Child with a Cleft Palate Saying 'six'

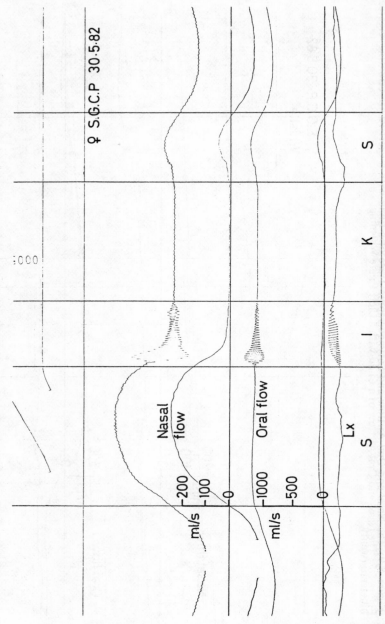

Figure 5.9: The Nasal and Oral Airflow and Laryngographic Trace of a Child with a Cleft Palate Counting 'eighteen, nineteen, twenty'

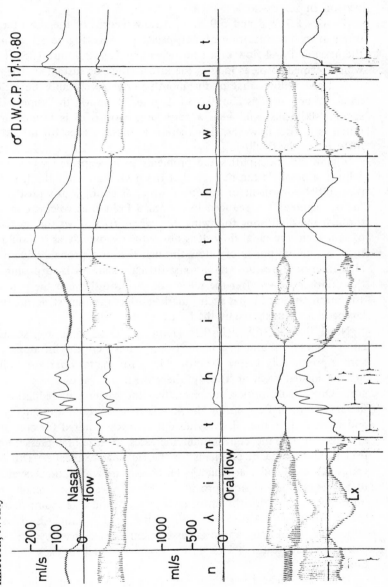

tion and subjective judgement of voice quality is, of course, to ascertain how good the agreement is between individual therapists and a large-scale survey in the UK has been completed (Razzell, Anthony and Watson, in preparation).

Figures 5.7, 5.8 and 5.9 show airflow records of the short-term or articulatory, modification of cleft-palate patients. Figure 5.7 is simply the nasal and oral flow of a child whistling. It lasts about 0.75 seconds which seemed to be as long as the effort could be sustained. The nasal flow trace follows that of the mouth fairly closely and the ratio of nasal to oral flow is about 0.35. Figure 5.8 shows the same patient saying 'six' /siks/ and here a very large ratio of 5 is found for the initial /s/. Note, however, that there is no nasal escape for the /k/ and little during the final /s/.

Figure 5.9 exemplifies the problems to be expected when a stop follows a nasal. It can be seen that the nasal flow after the first nasal (the initial consonant of 'nineteen' which is contiguous with the final /n/ of 'eighteen') is reduced in a normal fashion as voicing continues through the diphthong following, but where /t/ follows the medial /n/ of 'nineteen' the nasal flow does not reduce as quickly as it should and there is random oscillatory flow through the nose, probably due to the high inter-oral pressure and a 'loose-fitting' palate. It is surprising that this continues even after the release of the stop through the period of aspiration and that it has such a marked effect on some structure in the laryngeal area (as shown by the L_x trace).

Nasal flow is still high throughout the next nasal stop sequence ending 'nineteen' and beginning 'twenty' but here the intra-oral pressure is presumably below the critical level for palatal vibration. Following the medial nasal of 'twenty' there is again nasal escape during the stop. One should notice, however, that the patterns of reduction and increase in nasal flow during the vowels of this record are appropriate and normal. It is the relatively abrupt changes required for consonant articulation and the concomitant increases in intra-oral pressure that lead to these kind of problems for the cleft-palate speaker. This illustrates an essentially articulatory approach in which the waveforms of nasal and oral airflow provide, in specified contexts, quantitative information and insight into cleft-palate children's compensatory speech strategies (Anthony, 1980). This kind of analysis plays an important part in the approved assessment service given by the Cleft-palate Speech Research Unit in the Royal Hospital for Sick Children, Edinburgh.

There is a need for a simple portable unit for clinical use in the field which is capable of providing basic information on the presence and degree of nasal escape during speech. The system known as the Exeter Anemometer (Ellis, Flack, Curle and Selley, 1978; Ellis, 1979), consists of a sensing head made up of a thermistor mounted in a plastic nosemask. The thermistor is a sensitive detector of air temperature changes and the output from its amplifier unit is recorded on one track of a stereo cassette recorder; on the other is recorded the audio output of a microphone. A list of test words is read by the patient, the cassette is sent for processing and a hard-copy record is returned to the clinician.

Five kinds of velopharyngeal dysfunction have been identified by Netsell (1969) using intra-oral pressure and nasal flow. (1) A *gradual opening* dysfunction occurs when the speaker is able to achieve velopharyngeal closure at slower rates of utterance (repeated stop + vowel syllables were used as experimental tokens) with no nasal escape and adequate intra-oral air pressure, but nasal escape was detected and intra-oral pressure dropped at faster rates of utterance. (2) A *gradual closing* pattern was characterised by a gradual increase in intra-oral pressure as the syllable was repeated at faster rates (5 per second) with a corresponding decrease in nasal airflow, suggesting that dysfunction is apparent at the initiation of an utterance. However, the speaker is able to bring it under control as the utterance proceeds. (3) An *anticipatory opening* where the dysarthric speaker who was able to maintain closure during the utterance $/_\Lambda t_\Lambda d_\Lambda/$ produced two bursts of nasal airflow in the utterance $/_\Lambda t_\Lambda n_\Lambda/$, one for the /t/ and one for the /n/. Netsell suggests that the escape on /t/ is in anticipation of the later occurring /n/. (4) A *retentive opening* where the dysarthric speaker's production of $/_\Lambda n_\Lambda t_\Lambda/$ produces nasal escape on both consonants. Finally, with the relatively rare (5) *premature opening* where the speaker emits slight nasal escape during the first, and more pronounced nasal escape during the second consonant in an utterance like $/_\Lambda d_\Lambda t_\Lambda/$. The first occurs simultaneously with the increase in intra-oral air pressure and the second larger burst with the peak in intra-oral air pressure.

Netsell suggests that such information should be of value to the orthodontist in providing appropriate size of palatal lift for the patient with velopharyngeal dysfunction, and this application has been demonstrated by Hardy, Netsell, Schweiger and Morris (1969).

Figure 5.10 shows the inability of a Parkinson patient to sustain lung volume for adequate respiration during speech. Taking the upper level of the Functional Reserve Capacity (FRC) as zero one can see

Figure 5.10: The Respiration (Lung Volume) Record of a Parkinson Patient During Speech

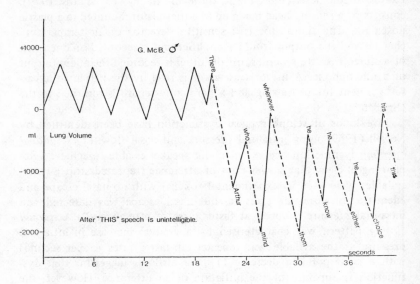

that the five cycles of quiet breathing, though of somewhat greater volume than one might have expected, are regular in frequency, have normal timing ratios and have their End Expiratory Levels near FRC. Expiration in the fifth cycle is not completed when an anticipatory inspiration is taken for the first Speech Breath Group, 'There — Arthur'. Speech takes the lung volume well down into the Expiratory Reserve Volume and the patient is not capable of the inspiratory effort required to raise lung volume again above FRC into the Inspiratory Reserve Volume. At the end of 'his — this', when speech has become unintelligible, no more is asked for and a number of Respiratory Recovery cycles (not shown) are taken by the patient to restore breathing to the initial pattern.

This long-term modification of airflow, or rather, change in lung volume, is also shown in the airflow record of a stammerer lasting about three minutes (Figure 5.11). Here one can see the long periods when no speech is produced and lung volume stays constant. During normal speech the timing and size of inspirations depend mainly on the style of speaking and the structure of the text, but in this example they occur at inappropriate intervals and are generally equal or greater

Figure 5.11: The Airflow Record of a Stammerer During Speech

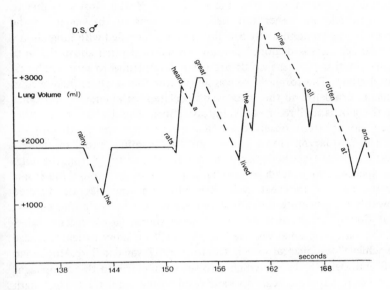

Source: Reprinted from Health Bulletin Vol. 36.6 by permission of the Controller, Her Majesty's Stationery Office.

than the volumes used immediately before. The result is that the lungs become inflated far beyond what is required, and lung volume is only restored to its normal level by expelling air at a high rate as End Volumes after the last two Speech Breath Groups.

There have been a number of airflow studies of dysphonia (Isshiki and von Leden, 1964; Yanagihara, 1967b; Yanagihara and von Leden, 1967; Kelman, Gordon, Simpson and Morton, 1975; Gordon, Morton and Simpson, 1978). Of particular interest from the perspective of this chapter is the work of Kelman *et al.* (1975) and Gordon *et al.* (1978) on the contribution of aerometry to making clinical decisions. Gordon *et al.* report on a series of 200 dysphonic patients who have been assessed using a combined airflow, laryngographic (see Chapter 4) and spectrographic (see Chapter 2) procedure. In mechanical dysphonia a large proportion of patients have a low air volume during phonation due to inadequate lung function and reduced respiratory effort. Nearly 80 per cent of patients with mechanical dysphonia in this study had problems in maintaining normal airflow rates. Two distinct patterns were observed. The first was characterised by an abnormally high flow rate with short phonation time and voice breaks due to inadequate glottal closure. In this type the inadequate glottal closure is due to cords which are either inflamed, oedematous or thickened. In the second type an abnormally low flow rate was coupled with long phonation time, increased glottal tension and habitual pitch above the optimum. In this type the cords are often bowed due to severe habitual vocal strain. The former type was most often found where there was an organic problem and the latter was associated with increased resistance in the glottis and reduced expiratory effort. The authors report that the various patterns observed served as a basis for successful therapy.

The post-laryngectomy patient presents a unique problem, namely that the vocal tract is deprived of its normal air supply from the lungs for speech, and instead air is breathed in and out through the stoma at the base of the neck wall. Rehabilitation strategies are directed towards reconnecting the supralaryngeal vocal tract to an air supply, and finding an alternative to the voicing source (for a recent review of the various alternatives, see Weinberg, 1981). Many patients manage to achieve 'oesophageal speech' (Stetson, 1937; van den Berg, Moollenar-Bijl and Damste, 1958) which involves taking air into the oesophagus in order to supply an egressive airstream to the vocal tract. The length of the Speech 'Breath' Cycle in oesophageal speech is severely restricted because the volumes of air that can be insufflated are much smaller, and average flow rates are much lower (Snidecor and Isshiki, 1965). Snidecor and Curry (1959) report that whereas a normal speaker produced an average of 12.54 words per inspiration in reading aloud, 'the oesophageal speaker averages 4.98 words per air change and has a much narrower range of performance'.

In a pilot study carried out recently at Queen Margaret College, Edinburgh, Phonetics Laboratory, an oesophageal speaker was asked to read the 'Exmoor' passage (see p. 86) while both stomal and nasal-oral airflow were monitored, using equipment similar to that described earlier (pp. 82–85). This speaker used 22 Speech Breath Cycles in reading the passage, as compared with the five used by the normal speaker. And some idea of the order of difference in average airflow rates can be gained from the fact that the oesophageal speaker expended a total of 96.5 ml of air through nose and mouth in reading the first sentence of the passage, as compared with the total of 435 ml expended by the normal speaker in reading the same sentence (see Table 5.1).

Discussion

The preceding analysis of the record above demonstrates why detailed information about the airflow characteristics of normal speech are necessary before any very significant statements even of a qualitative (as opposed to quantitative) nature, can be made about airflow in pathological speech. It is because the airflow patterns of normal speech cannot be accurately predicted from the conventional articulatory labels (e.g. 'voiced oral stop') given to speech sounds.

Imagine, for example, that examination of an airflow record from a dysarthric patient revealed a substantial oral flow during both nasal and oral stops. From a phonological point of view both of these segment classes imply a complete oral closure (i.e. are specified '+stop'). However, if the data from the normal speech analysed above are representative, then oral airflow during nasal stops must be deemed more significant, from a pathological point of view, than oral airflow during oral stops.

It may therefore be useful to attempt to summarise the evidence from this analysis concerning the greater or lesser importance of some of the phonetic features associated with the different classes of speech sounds in English.

Nasal flow is a vital element for nasal stops, although its onset and offset need not by any means coincide with the beginning and end of the segment, particularly in the neighbourhood of other sonorants. In sonorant segments the presence of nasal flow is more or less freely permitted. Conversely, zero nasal flow seems to be fairly important for obstruents. It is not always achieved, but certainly where the transition is from a nasal to an obstruent (or vice versa) the offset (or onset) of nasal flow is invariably much steeper. The explanation for this must be aerodynamic and physiological, since from an auditory standpoint one might have expected it to be the other way round (nasal resonance would be detectable in sonorant, rather than obstruent, sounds). The resistance of both fricatives and oral stops to the addition of nasal air flow is explained by the need to build up pressure in the oral cavity — to achieve turbulence in the first case, and an audible release in the second.

In oral stops the oral closure element appears to be particularly vulnerable. There are many instances of a quite considerable oral flow during a voiceless stop. The fact that many of these occur in the neighbourhood of /s/ suggests the possibility that greater ease of articulation may here dovetail nicely with phonological considerations. Despite the fact that there is oral flow during the 'stop', the [+ stop] vs. [− stop] contrast could be preserved by the much larger flow in the neighbouring fricative segment.

Voicing is a difficult feature to discuss in relation to variations in consonant production since voicing distinctions are more often conveyed by differences of relative timing than by properties of the segment itself. However, for nasal stops, where voicing does tend to be realised as an integral part of the segment, the evidence of the present data is that it may be vulnerable after a /s/, but is otherwise consistently achieved.

6 X-RAY TECHNIQUES

Martin J. Ball

Introduction

Unlike many of the other techniques described in this book, x-ray related techniques will not normally be readily available to the speech scientist or speech pathologist. There are, of course, straightforward reasons for this: in the wrong hands x-rays can be extremely dangerous; considerable training is necessary to learn how to operate the equipment which in turn is itself very complex and expensive. Therefore, anyone wishing to use an x-ray technique will probably only be able to do so indirectly — through the co-operation of the x-ray department of a hospital or similar research institution. This is not always an easy arrangement to make of course, though permission to use radiography with subjects suffering from a speech disorder is more readily given than to phoneticians pursuing purely theoretical problems.

The purpose of this chapter therefore is not to show the reader how to undertake an x-ray study personally, but rather to discuss the various x-ray techniques which are available and to help the reader decide which of these techniques would be most useful for any particular problem. It should also be noted at this stage that in the field of speech pathology, the major use of x-ray techniques is as an assessment and diagnostic tool, rather than as an aid to remediation.

X-Rays and their Properties

X-rays were discovered in 1895 by Professor W.C. Roentgen, and for this reason they are sometimes referred to as roentgen-rays. X-rays are in principle similar to rays of light or heat and radio waves, they are all classed as belonging to the electromagnetic spectrum (van der Plaats, 1969). The difference between the various rays in the spectrum is found in differences of frequency (the number of vibrations per second), although this can also be expressed as differences in the length of the wave — wavelengths being measured in divisions of a metre. For example, the wavelength of a radio transmission may be around 1km, whereas visible light lies between a range of 760 to 400nm (100nm = 0.001 mm), and x-rays have wavelengths below 0.5nm

(Ridgway and Thumm, 1968; van der Plaats, 1969), although 0.1nm is often considered the upper limit for x-rays in medical usage (see Figure 6.1).

Figure 6.1: The Electromagnetic Spectrum.

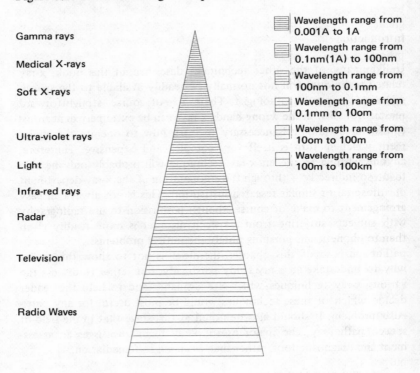

Gamma rays

Medical X-rays

Soft X-rays

Ultra-violet rays

Light

Infra-red rays

Radar

Television

Radio Waves

Wavelength range from 0.001A to 1A

Wavelength range from 0.1nm(1A) to 100nm

Wavelength range from 100nm to 0.1mm

Wavelength range from 0.1mm to 10om

Wavelength range from 10om to 100om

Wavelength range from 100m to 100km

Source: Courtesy of J. Ball.

X-rays are produced when electrons strike any solid body, and special *electron tubes* are used to achieve this. Design of the tubes differs according to whether a diagnostic or therapeutic (i.e. radiation therapy) function is required. The tube voltage will further decide whether the resultant rays will have a short wavelength, high x-ray energy and great penetration power (the so-called *hard x-rays*), or a longer wavelength, less x-ray energy and smaller penetration power (*soft x-rays*).

The major properties of x-rays of interest to the speech pathologist can be listed as follows (see Ridgway and Thumm, 1968; van der Plaats,

1969). First, x-rays are able to penetrate materials which would absorb and reflect visible light. This is of course their most useful property, and is reinforced by the fact that absorption does take place to some extent. This absorption (and in fact the scattering of the x-ray beam) is differential, by which it is meant that while all material is susceptible to penetration by x-rays, usually the more dense the material, the greater will be the absorption of the x-rays by that material. In this way it is possible to gauge density from x-rays films. A third important property showing the usefulness of x-rays is the fact that they travel in straight lines and are not easily refracted or reflected.

It is often necessary to have permanent records of x-ray information, and the following two properties are of importance here: x-rays affect photographic film in a similar way to visible light; and x-rays produce fluorescence (visible radiation) in certain materials. These aspects are further discussed below.

X-rays also have the property of producing ionisation in gases, which feature can be used to meter amounts of radiation. Radiation meters are of course important in ensuring that patients do not receive too great a degree of exposure to x-radiation. This leads to the last property of x-rays: they are able to damage or kill living cells. In radiation therapy this is of course a benefit, but in diagnostic work as in speech pathology, this is a danger to be avoided, and is the reason of course why access to x-ray equipment is so strictly vetted.

X-Ray Techniques

Although the general principles discussed above are common to all x-ray techniques, there are several different ways in which studies have been undertaken in the field of speech research, and it is the purpose of this section to outline the most important of these different techniques.

Perhaps the major choice facing the speech scientist in terms of x-ray techniques is that between still or cine film. (The distinction between direct and indirect radiography to be discussed below is to be found whether still or cine apparatus is used.) In terms of speech research — as speech is a serial activity — it has always been considered more appropriate to use x-ray cinematography (see Bladon and Nolan, 1977), although previous researchers have used still photography, often due to the dictates of circumstance, though it does have a value when non-dynamic aspects of the speech mechanism are under consideration. Taking x-ray cinematography as a general term covering all methods of moving x-ray film, we can follow Ridgway and Thumm

(1968) in their first major division between direct and indirect methods.

Direct. This area is also termed *radiography*. It is direct in the sense that the x-rays are recorded directly onto a photographic film or plate. For recording dynamic events *serial radiography* may be used. This involves the taking of a series of radiographs of the area concerned. Serial radiography can be as fast as 12 exposures per second. If the radiographs are reproduced on cinefilm the technique is termed *cineradiography*.

Indirect. This area is generally termed *fluorography*, because it involves the photography of a fluoroscopic screen. X-radiation falls onto the screen where it is converted into light energy. This light energy is proportional to the rate of absorption of the x-rays, so the various densities shown by the x-ray image, and the movements of the image in time are all reproduced on the screen. Still, serial and cine film may be used to record the screen of course, but the main drawback of fluorography is the low intensity of the image on the screen. This can be overcome by the use of an *image intensifier*. The most common type of image intensifier is a vacuum tube which converts the light image from the fluoroscopic screen into an electron image. The electrons are accelerated and re-converted into a smaller, brighter light image (Figure 6.2). Using

Figure 6.2: The Image Intensifier.

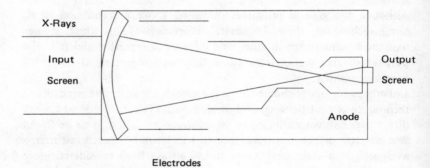

Source: Courtesy of J. Ball.

an image intensifier the resultant image may be recorded onto cine film, or more popularly these days, videotape. As Bladon and Nolan (1977) point out, video has the added advantages of live monitoring, instant playback and low x-ray dosage compared with other methods.

There are many specialist techniques using x-rays, and brief mention may be made of those relevant to speech science.

Panoramic Radiography. This is often used for dental purposes as it gives a complete picture of the upper and lower jaw in one picture, by employing a special x-ray tube which produces a wide beam.

Kymography. A technique used to show broad movements of internal organs (such as the heart). The method is explained more fully in van der Plaats (1969: p. 112), but will normally not give quite the amount of detail required by the speech scientist.

Tomography (or *Laminography, Planigraphy,* or *Stratigraphy*). This technique provides a cross-section of structures instead of a view of all planes. The x-ray source and the film are rotated in an arc in relation to the subject, and only that anatomic plane that has maintained the same distance from the source and the film will remain in focus. This method has been used extensively in speech research (particularly in larynx studies) but has the drawbacks of requiring a lot of film and a relatively high radiation dose. However, more recently, *computerised tomography* has overcome these drawbacks to some extent.

Xeroradiography. This method uses a special plate, which avoids the necessity of using a photographic chemical plate. Pictures may be obtained immediately, and the plate used again. This is particularly useful when ongoing monitoring of pictures is needed, though it does usually require a high radiation dosage. (Polaroid cameras are of course another way of accomplishing speed in obtaining pictures.) As Dicenta and Oliveras (1976) comment, xeroradiography is especially good at showing the relative densities of tissues.

Tracking. Techniques under this heading involve the tracking via x-ray film of objects attached to the vocal organs of the subject. From this information the movements of the organs of speech may be followed. Tracking has recently been combined with the use of *x-ray microbeams*, which is a recent development involving computer controlled low dosages of x-radiation. It is discussed further below.

It must be remembered that this section has only dealt with techniques likely to be of use to speech pathology and the speech sciences in general. Other techniques exist outside the scope of this chapter.

Radiographic Methods in Phonetics

Most x-ray studies conducted into speech have concentrated on the supra-glottal vocal tract. It is also the case that most studies have been conducted in profile, for as noted by Strenger (1968) x-ray photographs taken from the frontal position are often very difficult to interpret due to the dense mass of the bone of the lower jaw.

It is often desired to make particular structures stand out more clearly in the final photographs or film (especially the surface of the tongue), and for this reason various pastes are available (based on barium) with which the area in question may be coated. The attachment of lead pellets has also been undertaken for this purpose.

As Strenger (1968) reports, the *cephalostatic* x-ray study uses special equipment whereby the subject's head can be placed in an identical position each time recordings are being made — thus allowing easy comparison between the developed films.

A series of anatomical reference points, and lines derived from these (see Figure 6.3) are used where precise measurements are required, which measurements should be made from a single frame in the case of cine or video films. Strenger (1968) notes four areas where reasonably precise measurements may be obtained: the angle between the jaws, the movement of the upper and lower lips on the horizontal axis, the gap between the surfaces of the incisors, and the position and type of stricture between the tongue and the palate. Moll (1965) also notes that measurements can be made of velar height, tongue-pharynx distance and vocal fold opening; and Painter (1979) mentions larynx height.

A Review of Radiographic Studies in Phonetics

Right from the earliest days of the discovery of x-rays phoneticians have seen the great advantages of being able to see what is happening within the vocal tract where before they had had to rely upon educated guesswork. MacMillan and Keleman (1952) give a thorough review of phonetic studies using x-rays up until the 1940s, and it appears that the first paper on the subject was published in 1897, less than two years after Roentgen made his discovery.

The major concerns of the researchers in those early days were in perfecting x-ray techniques, and the studies of vowel and consonant production which they made were to some extent incidental. Much work went into finding a suitable way of marking the surface of the

Figure 6.3: A View of the Reference Points and Lines Necessary for a Phonetic Analysis of Articulation

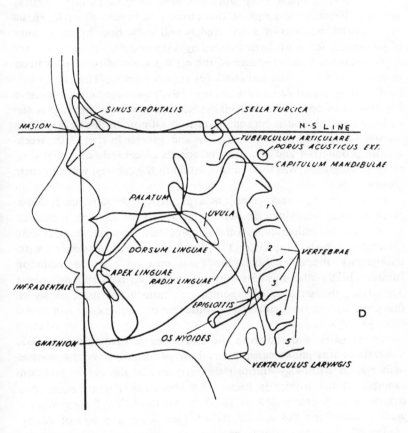

Source: Malmberg (1968).

tongue, and of ensuring that the position of the subject's head should remain constant. MacMillan and Kelemen (1952) comment that in its application to phonetics, the development of the x-ray technique 'shows periods of "spurts", with several important projects in progress simultaneously, alternating with periods of lull' (p. 685).

With the increasing use of cine and video-related techniques within the last twenty years or so, x-ray studies have become more popular among phoneticians as a way of studying speech, dispelling previous criticisms that still x-ray photographs were being used to explain dynamic events. Much x-ray work has been undertaken in phonetics, and it is beyond the scope of this chapter to review all of it. However, a brief mention of a few studies will show how broad an area of phonetic interest has been covered by x-ray studies.

As mentioned earlier, many of the early x-ray studies were involved in the perfection of the technique for speech research. This early work (reviewed in MacMillan and Kelemen, 1952) also contained phonetic description of course, in particular in relation to vowels, although some early studies did look at consonants as well. Of note in this field is work on the vowels of Spanish, Hungarian and French in the 1930s; work on the production and structure of vowels in general; and of course x-ray photography was used to help establish the cardinal vowel system (Jones, 1950).

More recently, x-radiography as a phonetic technique has found a place in some textbooks. In Malmberg (1968) for example a chapter is devoted to radiographic, palatographic and labiographic methods (Strenger, 1968); and Keller (1971) also has sections dealing with radiography and cineradiography. Final mention may be made of Painter (1979) who includes a short section on radiographic instrumentation, though it is disappointing to note a few inaccuracies in this contribution (particularly the confusion of radiography and fluoroscopy).

Recent work undertaken in the area tends to have either a purely phonetic and/or phonological motivation, or to have some connection with speech pathology through the provision of normative data. An example of the former is Balasubramanian (1981) who presented a straightforward description of Tamil vowels through still x-ray photographs. Sometimes this sort of study is carried out as a way of solving a phonetic or phonological problem or controversy. For example, Bladon and Nolan (1977) used videofluorography to ascertain the proportion of tongue tip to tongue blade alveolar sounds in English. Using videofluorography and cineradiography, Ball (1976) looked at the vowels of a northern dialect of Welsh to resolve a controversy about the production of the unrounded close central vowel phoneme. This information was also used to decide on a phonological description of the entire vowel system.

Studies having a connection with speech pathology tend to be normative investigations of specific speech areas to be used as comparisons for further pathological studies, or to be developments of new techniques which will be useful to speech pathology. In the former category, Subtelny, Oya and Subtelny (1972) can be mentioned. In this study ten normal speakers were examined through cineradiography producing sibilant phonemes (/s/ and /z/) within various phonetic environments. Considerable evidence on coarticulatory differences was collected with the specific aim of describing a normative framework for the treatment of defective sibilants in speech.

Other such normative studies include: Zawadski and Kuehn (1980) who examined the /r/ phoneme in American English (amongst several other researchers: see study for references); Hiroto (1980) who looked at vocal fold behaviour during phonation; Künzel (1979) who examined velum height and discusses the application of his technique to speech pathology; Iglesias, Kuehn and Morris (1980) who looked at movements of the pharynx wall and velum, again discussing the implications for speech pathology; and Fónagy (1976) who examined how emotion affects voice quality. Of particular relevance to the study of velopharyngeal insufficiency is research on the normative aspects of velar stretch and position (Mourino and Weinberg, 1975; Simpson and Colton, 1980; Seaver and Kuehn, 1980; Shaw, Folkins and Kuehn, 1980), and Weiss and Blackley's (1981) investigation with computerised tomography.

Finally, work on a particular new technique can be mentioned. Development has been taking place in Japan recently on a computer-controlled x-ray microbeam system for tongue-pellet tracking. Perhaps the best description of this is provided by Kiritani, Itoh and Fujimura (1975). The system involves tracking tongue movements by following small lead pellets affixed to its surface. The x-ray microbeams involved ensure a very low dosage of radiation. This technique has already been used in speech pathology, and this work will be discussed below.

X-Rays in Speech Pathology

Some of the more important and more recent research in the various areas of speech pathology that have used x-ray techniques will be reviewed in this section. Those areas of research which have used x-rays a great deal are reviewed before those which have used them less, though this does not necessarily imply that the techniques are best suited to any particular area.

Cranio-Facial Disorders

The term *cranio-facial disorder* is used here to cover the conditions *cleft palate* and *velopharyngeal insufficiency/inadequacy*.

It is perhaps not surprising that these areas of speech pathology have seen the greatest use of x-rays in research, due to the fact that treatment often involves medical attention, which in turn will usually necessitate the taking of x-rays. This section will review some of the studies undertaken with these disorders.

Moll (1965) in a contribution to the 1963 conference on cleft palate discusses the use of radiographic techniques in speech research with special emphasis on its role in cleft palate research. He divides x-ray techniques into three main types: still x-ray procedures, laminographic procedures and cineradiographic procedures; and his review refers to many important early studies. He concludes by noting five principles which apply to radiographic techniques in any area of speech research:

1. The technique should result in an accurate representation of structures.
2. It should place as few restraints as possible on the normal activity of the speech structures.
3. An adequate sampling of structural activity, preferably during connected speech, should be provided.
4. The technique should provide for correlating individual pictures with particular speech segments.
5. Film analysis procedures which result in accurate, quantitative data should be used. (Moll, 1965: p. 138)

Similarly, one of the classic text books on cleft palate (Grabb, Rosenstein and Bzoch, 1971) devotes a chapter (Williams, 1971) to radiographic methods in the analysis of cleft palate speech, along with many other passing references to the subject elsewhere in the volume. The aim of Williams in his chapter is to 'show how research in defining normal velo-pharyngeal closure using radiographic techniques has clinical applications in diagnosis and treatment' (p. 767), and he presents a review of past studies and different techniques. He discusses the problem of standardisation in the analysis of radiographic evidence, but concludes that such evidence has been of value in surgical and prosthetic rehabilitation and in diagnosis.

Many studies have been undertaken using radiographic techniques in the field of cranio-facial disorders and of course it will not be possible to review all of them. However a study of the literature reveals various areas of specific interest. First there is the use of x-ray techniques as a straightforward description of a particular disorder, or as a diagnostic tool. An example of the former is found in Shprintzen, Croft, Berkman and Rakoff (1980) who used videofluoroscopy and endoscopy to study patients suffering from the facio-auriculo-vertebral malformation complex. They discovered that while over half of the patients suffered from velopharyngeal insufficiency, only two out of these twelve actually had cleft palate.

In terms of a diagnostic study, Bowman and Shanks (1978) used cephalometry to study a group of patients with suspected velopharyngeal insufficiency. Looking at radiographs of the /i/ and /s/ phonemes, they concluded that the former gave a better indication of the presence of insufficiency.

A second group of studies is concerned with comparisons between disordered subjects and normals. This is usually in terms of the description of a particular physiological feature, for example Glaser, Skolnick, McWilliams and Shprintzen (1979) compared the dynamics of Passavant's ridge in normal subjects and those with velopharyngeal insufficiency using videofluoroscopy; whereas Zwitman, Gyepes and Ward (1976) examined velar and lateral wall movements.

A third important area is the assessment of subjects post-operatively. Kuehn and Van Demark (1978) assessed velopharyngeal competency following a teflon pharyngoplasty. Pre- and post-operative x-ray information suggested considerable improvement in competency in the first three months following the operation. Lewis and Pashayan (1980) examined the effects of pharyngeal flap surgery on twenty patients and found that lateral pharyngeal wall movement had not improved in these cases. Finally, in a slightly different area, Enany (1981) examined the effects of primary osteoplasty in unilateral cleft lip and palate subjects.

Fourthly, the area of longitudinal studies of child development has attracted much work. The use of metal implants trackable by x-rays is often found to provide detailed information on growth patterns in subjects suffering from a variety of cranio-facial disorders. However, these studies rarely include direct reference to speech disorders.

Lastly, there are those studies concerned with evaluating different investigative techniques in the context of cranio-facial disorders. For example, Williams and Eisenbach (1981) compare still x-radiography with cinefluorography in a study of velopharyngeal insufficiency. The authors conclude that 'one is apt to misdiagnose the presence or absence of velopharyngeal insufficiency on the order of 30% of the time when relying on the lateral still x-ray technique alone' (p. 45). This is attributed to the limited speech sample that can be used in still filming as opposed to cine.

Zwitman, *et al*. (1976) compared cineradiography with endoscopy. In this particular instance the radiographic technique was used to assess the accuracy of endoscopy in the examination of velar and lateral wall movement. The authors found that cineradiography confirmed endoscopic observation in a larger percentage of patients.

Shelton and Trier (1976) discuss the use of cinefluorography in the measurement of velopharyngeal closure, and conclude that measures in addition to fluorography are needed, and a comparison of various measure types is provided.

Laryngeal Disorders

This section will review some of the work done on disorders of the larynx resulting in voice disorders, including such areas as vocal fold tension, laryngeal disease and laryngectomy.

From quite early on the advantages of x-ray techniques in the study of laryngeal disorders have been recognised. In one of the major textbooks on voice (Luchsinger and Arnold, 1965) a whole section is included on the use of radiographic methods in voice analysis. The section reviews various suitable techniques (e.g. kymography, fluoroscopy, tomography and cineradiography), and references to many of the pioneering studies in the application of x-ray techniques to voice may be found, particularly the use of tomography. Many of these studies were concerned with normal voice characteristics, but van den Berg (1955) is mentioned for his cineradiographic study of the production of oesophageal pseudovoice.

Another study concerned with oesophageal voice is DeSantis *et al*. (1979). They note that sometimes the attempt to introduce oesophageal voice to laryngectomy patients fails, and state that other research has shown the importance of the cervical portion of the oesophagus in the production of oesophageal voice. Their investigation concerns the advantages and disadvantages of various radiographic techniques in the study of this area.

Ward *et al*. (1979) compare various techniques in the study of laryngeal disease. Computerised tomography appeared to the authors to be the clearest technique for showing tumors, cystic lesions and traumatic lesions. There were reduced radiation doses, and the technique was cheaper to use, also eliminating the need for conventional tomography or laryngography. (See also Pahn, 1981, for an x-ray diagnosis method for superior laryngeal nerve palsy.)

Pruszewicz, Obrebowski and Gradzki (1976) used both tomography and lateral radiography to examine the larynxes of several groups of patients undergoing different drug treatments. Voice quality in the patients had been affected, with a generally lowered pitch, smaller pitch range, shortened phonation time and a tendency to tire easily. The study showed an increase of calcification of the larynx cartilages and an asymmetry of the vocal folds and related structures.

Ardran and Kemp (1967) used tomography and radiography in a study of the function of the larynx following the King-Kelly operation involving the lateral fixation of a vocal cord in patients suffering from bilateral vocal cord palsy. The x-ray pictures clearly show pre- and post-operative conditions, and are compared with previous work undertaken by the same authors on normal vocal cord activity.

These studies are representative of the sort of work done in the general area of laryngeal disorders, but more recently a new technique based on xeroradiography has been developed, and this has been applied to many types of voice disorder (MacCurtain, 1981; Berry *et al.,* 1982a). The full name of this new development is *Xeroradiography-Electro-Laryngography* (XEL), and it encompasses a joint use of xeroradiography with the electrolaryngograph (see Chapter 4). This produces simultaneous information on soft tissue changes in the vocal tract in terms of a visual display of the Lx and Fx waves on the electrolaryngograph, and the xeroradiographic picture. One of the advantages claimed for the technique is that in most cases the need for direct laryngography is eliminated.

This particular technique has been developed to be used easily in the clinic, and for this purpose the reading of the xeroradiographs is facilitated through the drawing up of a set of 17 voice quality parameters, easily located on the xeroradiograph (see Figure 6.4). This technique is concerned with both diagnosis and treatment, though it should be noted that the xeroradiographic aspect is mostly helpful for diagnosis.

A representative study using XEL is found in Ranford (1982). Evidence is presented from XEL to show the nature of a voice disorder in a patient that had previously been undiagnosed. The xeroradiographs (see Figures 6.5 and 6.6) seemed to show a loss of smoothness in the vocal fold vibration and some tilting of the laryngeal assembly in phonation due to an imbalance of muscle activity. Figure 6.7 shows a xeroradiograph of the same patient after treatment. (See also Berry *et al.*, 1982a, b for investigations of normal and disordered voice.)

Figure 6.4: Anatomical Parameters used in XEL Listed in Order of Frequency of Use in Analysing Voice Disorders

1. vocal folds
2. laryngeal airway
3. ventricular folds
4. laryngopharynx
5. vestibule of the larynx
6. epiglottis
7. vallecula
8. oropharynx
9. hyoid bone
10. hypopharynx
11. thyroid cartilage
12. length of vocal tract
13. cricothyroid vizor
14. nasopharynx
15. retropharygeal soft tissue
16. tongue gesture

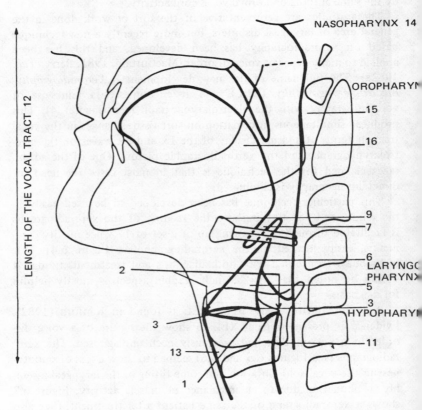

Source: Reprinted with permission from Berry *et al*. (1982). Courtesy of F. MacCurtain.

Figure 6.5: Xeroradiograph Taken at Rest

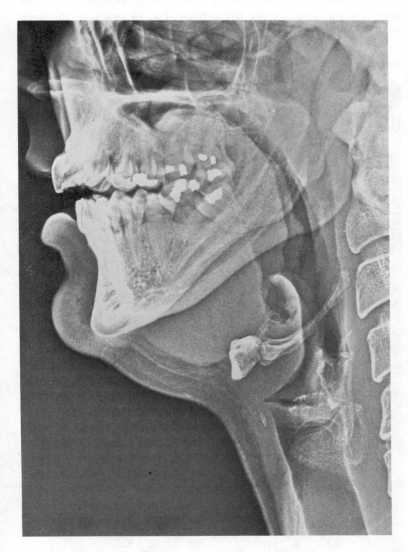

Source: Courtesy of H.J. Ranford.

Figure 6.6: Xeroradiograph Before Therapy. During [i:] the vocal folds are displaced upwards due to increased muscle activity bringing the thyroid cartilage nearer the hyoid bone. The air spaces of the laryngopharynx are measurably reduced by constriction of the extrinsic laryngeal muscles. Convolutions along the tongue root also indicate increased tension.

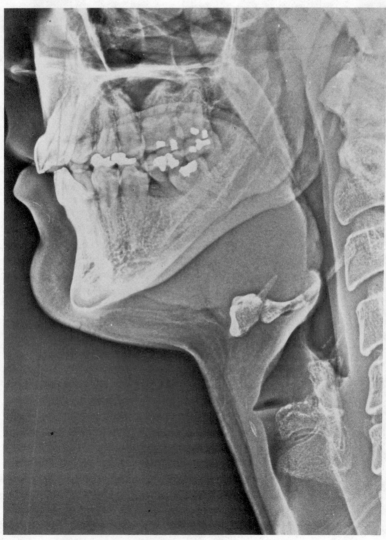

Source: Courtesy of H.J. Ranford.

Figure 6.7 Xeroradiograph After Nine Month's Therapy. The larynx is lowered during production of [i:] when compared with Figure 6.6. The air spaces of the laryngopharynx have opened up to act as a more effective resonating chamber for the voice. Also the tongue root is noticeably smoother, indicating less tension.

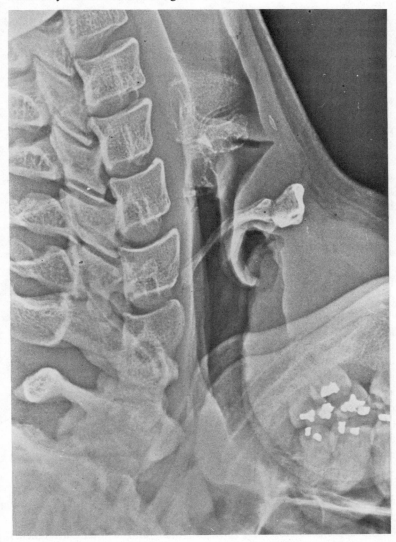

Source: Courtesy of H.J. Ranford.

The development of XEL, bringing together two of the techniques described in this book, is a very interesting step forward for speech pathologists; for it brings a very sophisticated diagnostic ability within the reach of the clinic.

Stuttering

A series of recent publications will be examined that show the value that x-ray techniques could be in the area of stuttering. Zimmerman (1980a, b, c) used high-speed cinefluorography to examine articulation in stutterers. In the first of the three studies he examined the speech of six stutterers in comparison with seven normal speakers. The passages that were recorded from all the speakers on this occasion contained only speech that was perceptually fluent. The aim was to describe the movement of the articulators in terms of space and time, and to see what differences there were if any between stutterers and normals during what appeared to be fluent speech. The second investigation used the same technique to look at a group of stutterers comparing their fluent and non-fluent utterances. The third study seeks to combine information gained from the previous two to propose a model of disfluency.

The results obtained in the first study suggested that stutterers and normal speakers differ in how speech production is organised even in speech which appears fluent perceptually. These differences manifested themselves in consistently longer durations between movement onsets, achievements of peak velocity, and voice onsets for the stutterers in comparison with the normals. Zimmerman (1980a) also reported that the stutterers showed 'longer steady state positioning for the lip and jaw during vowel production and a greater asynchrony between lip and jaw movement' (p. 95). The stutterers' utterances were also of longer duration than the normals'. Zimmerman feels that an explanation for these findings could be found in terms of compensatory behaviour. He notes that 'reducing the amount of movement (displacement) and/or increasing the duration of a production might allow the stutterer to gain better control of the motor output' (Zimmerman, 1980a: p. 106). However he concludes by warning about generalisations being made from such a small subject population.

The second investigation utilised the same x-ray technique on four male stutterers in comparison with one female non-stutterer. The results of this study showed that articulator relationships occurred in the speech of stutterers (both in fluent and disfluent utterances) that were not usually found in normal speakers, and that 'a systematic repositioning [of articulators] occurs preceding the release from oscillatory or tonic (posturing) behaviors' (p. 117). Zimmerman notes that the most frequent of these relationships involved lowering of the jaw, reshaping of the tongue towards the rest position, and lowering of the lower lip. Zimmerman suggests that some of these effects can be accounted for by reflex interactions among the muscles of articulation: 'imbalances in afferent-efferent interactions among brainstem structures' (p. 119).

The author feels that these conclusions have direct implications for therapy, 'therapy might be geared to putting the system back in balance' (p. 119), and he quotes as an example, 'instead of dealing with relaxation of the lip muscles when they are involved in oscillatory behaviors, jaw closers might advantageously be relaxed' (p. 119). The author concludes by noting that further work in the area of generalised and muscle specific relaxations seems justified.

Zimmerman (1980c) proposes a model of stuttering as a disorder of movement, drawing on information from the first two studies. He suggests that the movement of articulators in time and space (and the interactions between articulators) operate within a permissible range of variability. When this range is exceeded for whatever reason, the articulatory system is thrown out of balance, resulting in oscillatory behaviour or static positioning (stuttering and blocking). Further research is suggested, as only the movement patterns of the upper articulators have been studied.

Zimmerman's work has shown how x-ray techniques can add much to our knowledge of articulatory behaviour in stuttering and in the theoretical consideration of this problem. One other study can be briefly mentioned here: Fujita (1966) who, as part of an examination into the role of phonation in stuttering, took posterior-anterior x-rays of one Japanese stutterer. He reported irregular or inconsistent opening and closing of the pharyngolaryngeal cavity and asymmetric tight closure of the pharyngeal cavity. Again, there are obvious drawbacks in this study from the small subject population.

Aphasia, Apraxia, Dysarthria

Some x-ray studies have been undertaken in this area of speech pathology, though it has not proved as popular a technique as in the field of cranio-facial disorders for instance.

In the case of dysarthria, Kent and Netsell (1975) conducted cine-radiographic and spectrographic investigations into the speech of an ataxic dysarthric. They found abnormalities in speaking rate, stress patterns, articulatory placements, velocities of articulator movements and fundamental frequency contours; and they conclude, 'perhaps ... ataxic dysarthria is characterized by a generalized hypotonia ...' (p. 129), this hypotonia resulting in the slowness of movement that was observed.

Hirose, Kiritani, Ushijima and Sawashima (1978) used the x-ray microbeam system to analyse abnormal articulatory movements in two dysarthric patients − the first an ataxic dysarthric of cerebellar origin, the second a case of amyotrophic lateral sclerosis. Different patterns of articulator movement were recorded, with additional evidence provided by electromyography. The authors feel that this sort of study is a 'promising approach for elucidating the nature of central problems of speech production and for a differential diagnosis of various types of dysarthrias' (p. 96). The same technique is employed by Hirose *et al.* (1981) in a study of dysarthric movements in patients with Parkinsonism.

An x-ray microbeam investigation was also employed in a study of apraxia (Itoh *et al.*, 1980). The authors found that temporal organisation among the articulators was disturbed, and also that the 'pattern and velocity of the articulator movements of the patient ... were different from those of typical dysarthric patients' (p. 66).

In the field of aphasia x-rays in the form of tomography have been used as a diagnostic tool to locate the position of lesions in the brain. However this use of x-rays is more properly described as medical than as part of speech pathology, and is therefore not within the scope of this chapter.

Other Disorders

X-ray techniques have also been used in other areas of speech pathology, though to a lesser extent. Various studies have been undertaken in the area of articulation. To understand better the role of proprioceptive feedback, Putnam and Ringel (1976) investigated articulation in subjects with temporarily induced oral-sensory deprivation, finding a loss of precision in lip, tongue and jaw movements. Kuehn and Tomblin (1977) looked at child speech in the specific area of /w/ - /r/ substitutions. Their findings suggested that while the subjects were 'possibly differentiating between /w/ and intended /r/, ... the articulatory target configurations appeared to be nondiscriminatory' (p. 462), and that systematic lip, jaw and tongue differences were required successfully to discriminate the two sounds.

Also in the field of articulation, studies have been done on articulation problems involving dental and oral surgery. Zimmerman, Kelso and Lander (1980) and Shelton, Furr, Johnson and Arndt (1975) discuss two such cases.

X-ray studies have also been undertaken in the field of hearing problems. For example, Seaver, Andrews and Granata (1980) discuss velar positioning in hearing-impaired adults and conclude that the hypernasality found in the hearing impaired is of a different character to that found in cleft-palate patients. Bergstrom (1978) discusses the differences between congenital and acquired deafness in cleft-palate patients.

Clinical Applications

The above review has shown the versatility of radiographic techniques in speech pathology, both as a general research tool to aid our understanding of different disorders, but also as a method of diagnosis. In terms of its clinical applications, the diagnostic ability of the techniques is of primary importance. X-ray techniques as they have been defined here play no direct role in treatment (radiotherapy is outside the scope of this chapter), though of course accurate diagnosis is in itself a pre-requisite to effective treatment.

As the review has shown, radiography can play an important role in the diagnosis of various cranio-facial disorders, voice disorders, dysarthrias and so on, and that different techniques are suitable for different areas. However, the major problem of accessibility remains. Comparatively few speech pathologists have ready access to these techniques, though the XEL project in Britain promises well for the assessment of laryngeal disorders.

Other problems remain in assessing the usefulness of radiography to the clinician. Returning to Moll's (1965) five principles, it might be argued that in many cases accurate film analysis is not made, and that the technique can become too invasive — through the introduction of barium paste on the tongue, lead pellets or other marking devices, thereby going against Moll's principle of placing as few restraints as possible on normal speech activity. There are also of course the dangers from radiation to consider, even though recent developments do seem to have minimised these.

In view of these considerations, what alternative techniques could be employed to give similar information without the drawbacks? Two techniques that have been used in speech research to give pictorial information of articulator movement are *fibroscopy* and *ultrasonics*. A fibrescopic analysis involves the insertion of the fibrescope via the oral or nasal cavities to observe the speech mechanism. Evidence from the fibrescope is photographed (still or cine) for a permanent record. An example of a fibrescopic investigation of an apraxic subject is given in Itoh, Sasanuma and Ushijima (1979). A later study by Itoh *et al*. (1980, reviewed above) concluded that x-radiography gave clearer results, and it must be acknowledged that fibroscopy is a very invasive technique.

Ultrasonic techniques are also invasive, in that an ultrasonic probe is fitted within the vocal tract, and the echoes received help to delineate the shapes of the articulators. Niimi and Simada (1980) report an experiment where ultrasonics was used to describe the frontal section of the tongue, an area which has been difficult to observe radiographically.

Finally *stroboscopy* can be mentioned. This technique is mostly used in voice investigations, where a stroboscopic light source combined with a laryngeal mirror can give information as to the frequency of vocal cord vibration. This method is however not very sophisticated, and its limitations are fully discussed in Luchsinger and Arnold (1965).

Conclusion

It would appear that as a technique for investigating the speech mechanism, radiography is difficult to equal in the provision of visual information. As a clinical diagnostic tool for the *speech pathologist* the potential advantages are seldom realised however. It would seem important therefore not only to continue research with x-rays into all kinds of speech and language disorders, but to develop easier access to and fuller provision of radiographic techniques for speech pathologists.

Acknowledgement

My thanks to Jennifer Ball for designing Figures 6.1 and 6.2.

7 DELAYED AUDITORY FEEDBACK

Chris Code

Introduction

In the normal individual, speech sounds are fed back to the inner ear via air (air-conducted feedback) and bone (bone-conducted feedback) with a delay of about 0.001 seconds (Yates, 1963). Delayed auditory feedback (DAF), or delayed sidetone, involves extending the time between the utterance of a speech sound and its auditory perception.

The DAF effect on a normal speaker, first described by Lee (1950a, b), is characterised by a number of alterations to normal speech which Fairbanks (1955) described as the *indirect* and the *direct* effects of DAF. The indirect effects are reduction in rate of speech, increase in intensity and increase in fundamental frequency. According to Fairbanks, these indirect effects are due to the subject's efforts to overcome the influence of the DAF. The direct articulatory effects which are observed include repetition of syllables and continuants, mispronunciations, omissions, substitutions, additions and omitted word endings. Lee (1950a) referred to the DAF effect as 'artificial stuttering'.

Achieving delays in auditory feedback is essentially uncomplicated and can be accomplished with a good standard reel-to-reel tape recorder with separate record and playback heads. The subject's speech is recorded on the tape via the record head, the tape passes to the playback head and the speech fed back to the subject through headphones. The delay in auditory feedback is determined by a combination of the distance between the heads and the speed of the tape. For example, an inter-head gap of 1.25 inches over a tape speed of 7.5 in/s will give a delay of about 160 ms. Four delay times (80, 160, 330, and 660 ms) are therefore available from such a tape recorder with the four tape speeds 1.875, 3.75, 7.5, and 15 in/s.

More delay times are available with a tape recorder that has either a moveable record or playback head, and Tiffany, Hanley and Sutherland (1954) and Huggins (1967) describe different devices for converting tape recorders in such a way that a large variety of accurate delay times can be achieved. The device described by Huggins utilises a

Figure 7.1: A Simple Device for Varying the Length of the Tape Path on a Standard Tape Recorder

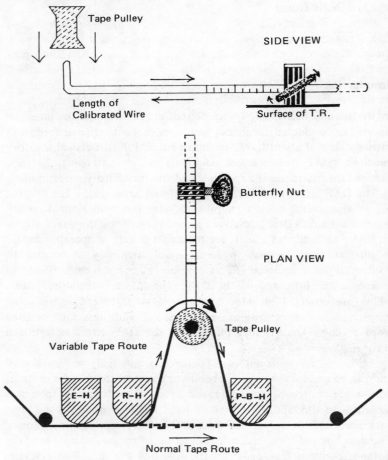

Source: Reprinted with permission from Code (1979). Courtesy of E. LeGin.

micrometer bolted to the surface of a tape recorder which can be adjusted to vary the length of the tape path between the heads. The device has the advantage that it does not involve moving heads and the tape recorder can still be used in the normal way when not required for DAF. An even simpler method is described by Code (1979) for varying the length of the tape path (Figure 7.1). All that is required is a tape pulley, a length of wire about 1 mm thick and a clamping screw that can hold the wire and allow adjustment. The clamping screw can be bolted to the upper surface of the tape recorder and the length of wire can be calibrated.

Both Butler and Galloway (1957) and Siegel, Fehst, Garber and Pick (1980) describe a versatile method for obtaining a range of delay times employing two tape recorders arranged in series. The subject's speech is delayed on one recorder and then fed to the other where the delay produced by the first recorder is combined with the delay chosen on the second. This method can provide a range of delay times depending on the tape speeds and inter-head gaps available on the machines.

Figure 7.2: The Aberdeen Speech Aid Solid-state DAF Device. The bench and pocket model are shown.

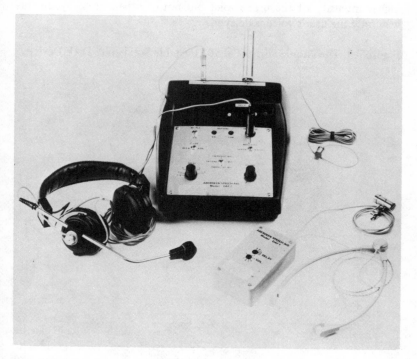

Source: Courtesy of Aleph One, Cambridge, England.

Apart from using standard tape recorders there are a number of commercially produced machines available. The 'Phonic Mirror' is a multiple-head tape machine (one record and five playback heads) which employs a tape loop. This machine gives a range of five delay times (50, 100, 150, 200 and 250 ms). With recent developments in silicon chip technology a number of tapeless, solid-state devices, which achieve delays electronically, have become available. The Aberdeen Speech Aid (Low and Lindsay, 1979) is a device developed in Britain which comes in two models. The larger desk model is for clinical and laboratory use and the pocket size model (10 X 5 X 2.5 cm) is for personal use and includes a lapel microphone and earphones (Figure 7.2). The device provides continuous delay from 30 to 300 ms, and is capable of binaural and mononaural presentation of DAF. It gets over the problem of delaying the voices of others close to the user by employing a switch which is activated by the higher intensity of the user's voice but not of others close by. In this way only the user's voice is delayed.

Figure 7.3: The Phonic Mirror PM 505 Portable Solid-state DAF Device

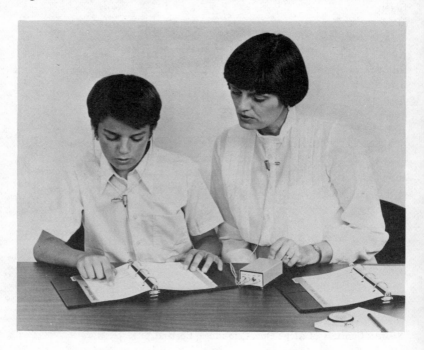

Source: Courtesy of Phonic Mirror International, Copenhagen.

The Danish Phonic Mirror PM 505 (Figure 7.3) is a similar device slightly larger than the Aberdeen Speech Aid (11 X 6.4 X 3.8 cm), and provides continuous delays from 25 to 220 ms. It also employs a lapel microphone and earphones. The Dystech 1000 is a body-worn DAF device developed recently in the United Sates and briefly described by Muellerleile (1981).

Delayed Auditory Feedback in Normal Speakers

There is variability in the degree of disruption experienced by different groups of normal speakers under DAF. Chase, Sutton, First and Zubin (1961) found that children between 4 and 6 years show less disturbance of speech than older children between 7 and 9 years under a delay of 200 ms.

Mackay (1968) tested the same age groups as Chase *et al.* (1961) with a variety of delay times. He found that the delay required to produce disruption in speech decreases with age. Children in the younger group (4-6 years) showed maximum disturbance under a delay of 500 ms, whereas children in the older group (6-9 years) experienced peak disruption at 400 ms, delay. In addition, Mackay reports that the disturbances of the younger group were more severe than those of the older group, which were in turn more severe than the disruptions observed in an adult group (20-26 years). In agreement with most other studies, Mackay also reports that 200 ms is the delay which produces maximum disruption in adults.

Work by Buxton (1969) and recently Siegel *et al.* (1980) tends to confirm Mackay's findings. Moreover, Buxton found that the most disruptive delay-time for older adults between 60 and 81 years was 400 ms. It therefore appears that the maximumly disruptive delay time decreases with age from 500 ms in early childhood, to 400 ms in later childhood, and to 200 ms in adults, where some kind of peak is reached. It then increases with old age to 400 ms. It also appears that the disruption caused by DAF becomes more pronounced with age which suggests that there is a reduction in reliance on auditory feedback with increasing age (Siegel *et al.*, 1980).

The relationship between sex differences and DAF is less clear. Mahaffey and Stromsta (1965) found that the optimum delay for male subjects was in the region of 180 ms, where the optimum delay which produced the most disruption for female subjects was 270 ms, Timmons and Boudreau (1972) report that when delays of 0 to 500 ms were presented in random order to male and female subjects no differences in reactions were observed, but differences do emerge when the delay times are compared in order of their presentation. However, Buxton (1969), in his study of sex differences, found no differences at all. Those studies that have found differences tend to indicate that males are more vulnerable to DAF than females.

It seems to be generally established that more fluent and rapid speakers show less disruption under DAF (Beaumont and Foss, 1957; Mackay, 1968; Buxton, 1969). Mackay found that the slower a subject's speech was without DAF the more disruption of speech occurred under DAF. This correlation was observed in all the age groups that Mackay investigated — young children, older children and adults. Conversely, Buxton found that naturally rapid speakers show less disturbance in their speech under delays ranging from 100 to 600 ms. Furthermore, evidence indicates that a rapid speaker requires a shorter delay time to produce maximum instability whereas naturally slow speakers show maximum disruption under longer delay times.

In summary, there are individual differences in reactions to DAF by normal speakers. Some speakers are comparatively unaffected while others show severe distortions of fluency, vocal pitch and intensity. Disturbances in speech appear to decrease with age with adults being less affected than children. However, older adults are more affected than younger adults. There is some evidence that male subjects show more disturbance than female subjects and more rapid fluent speakers are less affected than less rapid and less fluent speakers.

The Role of Delayed Auditory Feedback in Speech Science

The main thrust of research into the DAF effect with normal speakers has been the examination of the role of auditory feedback in speech production. Explanations for the DAF phenomenon abound (see Code, 1980 for further discussion). Lee (1950a) was among the first to propose a model of speech production which took account of the effect. The model is made up of feedback loops which are approximately proportional in length to the time necessary to perform the speech activity associated with the particular loop. Four hierarchically arranged loops make up the model: an articulatory loop (phonemes), a voice loop (syllables), a word loop and a thought loop. It is the shorter loops — articulatory and voice — which are affected by DAF. An important property of the model is that any unit may be repeated if monitoring is dissatisfied with the first performance, and there is a common junction for all the loops which represents a cortical speech centre. Lee suggests, therefore, that stuttering and 'artificial' stuttering result from a disfunction or instability of closed-loop feedback at the phonemic and/or syllabic level.

Cherry and Sayer (1956) conducted a classic series of experiments using white masking noise with 54 severe stutterers and were able to show that intense auditory feedback masking resulted in almost complete fluency. They found, however, that band-pass filtering of the white noise to allow only high frequencies above 500Hz through to the speaker, reduced stuttering; whereas filtering to allow only low frequencies below 500Hz, did not reduce dysfluency. The authors conclude that stuttering must be related to an individual's perception of their own low frequency, bone-conducted, feedback that produces instability in a closed-loop feedback system.

The model of speech production proposed by Fairbanks (1954) which accounts for the DAF effect includes a comparator to which auditory, tactile and proprioceptive information is fed back via a sensor unit. These signals are compared to output and a calculation is performed by the comparator to determine discrepancies between the two signals.

This model, like Lee's, is dominated by auditory feedback and assumes closed-loop control. Contemporary phonetics considers that an entirely automatic closed-loop model or an entirely open-loop model, with no feedback control, cannot explain all that is now known about speech production. It is also established that auditory feedback is far too slow to achieve *ongoing* monitoring and correction of articulatory events. Auditory feedback can only be post-event in its influence on the control of speech production. For ongoing closed-loop control, proprioceptive feedback via the gamma-loop system of the muscle spindles appears to hold the best promise (see Hardcastle, 1976, for further discussion), and some theoretical predictive *feedforward* capabilities of the central nervous system have been proposed (see Borden, 1979, for comprehensive review).

Borden, Dorman, Freeman and Niimi (1976) examined the electromyographic (EMG) performance of normal speakers under DAF and found EMG activity associated not only with the dysfluent speech produced, but also with aborted articulatory attempts. The study concludes that the DAF effect is due to a conflict between proprioceptive feedback providing information to proceed and auditory feedback providing information to wait. Borden (1979) also points out that EMG data taken while subjects are under DAF is characteristically inconsistent, indicating an intermittent attentiveness to the auditory signal on the part of the speaker rather than true closed-loop error correction.

Applications in Speech Pathology and Therapeutics

There have been a number of studies in speech pathology and therapeutics employing the paradigm of DAF. Most of this research has been into stuttering, although there have been recent developments in DAF research with aphasic, apraxic and dysarthric patients.

Stuttering

While the DAF effect on normal speakers is generally a negative disruption of the normal speech pattern, interference with auditory feedback in stutterers can have surprisingly positive effects upon fluency (Webster and Lubker, 1968; Van Riper, 1973). But where it is the more fluent normal speaker who reacts less to DAF, in the case of stutterers it has been shown that it is the more severe who respond most positively (Soderberg, 1969; Van Riper, 1971).

While the critical delay time for producing maximum disruption in normal speakers is fairly well established, there appear to be more individual differences amongst stutterers with regard to critical delay times for producing improvements in fluency. Lotzmann (1961) reported that varying the delay around 50 ms, produced a marked reduction in blocks, and in all cases in the sample he studied the optimum delay times were shorter than the delays used to produce dysfluency in normal speakers. For an individual stutterer who benefits from DAF there is probably a critical delay time which produces maximum fluency, probably a relatively short delay time; and a separate critical delay time which produces maximum dysfluency, probably a longer delay time.

The Relationship Between Genuine and Artificial Stuttering

It is a common observation that stuttering is often at its worse in the initiation of utterances where auditory feedback does not come into play. This observation is not consistent with a perceptual theory of stuttering, although this is not to say that auditory feedback does not play some part in stuttering. It is clear, for instance, that DAF and perhaps to a greater extent auditory feedback masking, can have a beneficial effect upon the speech of stutterers, which is more than mere 'distraction'. If DAF was simply acting as a distraction, then *any* delay-time would produce fluency. The same goes for auditory masking. For masking to eliminate dysfluency, it must be the low bone-conducted frequencies which are masked.

It is also clear that DAF causes a sort of 'artificial' stuttering in normal speakers. However, there is evidence to suggest that the two phenomena are mediated by separate mechanisms. Neelly (1961) found that the characteristics were different and amount of adaption to DAF was different between stutterers and normal speakers, and in a perceptual study listeners were able to distinguish successfully between the speech of stutterers and normal speakers under DAF. Code (1979) was able to provide some support for Neelly's view that stuttering and artificial stuttering are separate phenomena in a study which compared the EMG signals taken from the upper lip of a severe stutterer without DAF and a normal speaker made dysfluent by DAF. An analysis of the amplitudes and durations of the EMG signals revealed that there were significant differences in the muscular activity of the two subjects. However, EMG data taken while the stutterer was reading fluently under low frequency (below 500Hz) masking, and while the non-stutterer was reading normally without DAF showed that there were no significant differences in muscular activity, indicating that muscular activity in masking-induced fluency in stutterers cannot be differentiated from muscular activity in normal fluency using EMG. This last finding supports a similar one by Dewar, Dewar and Anthony (1976). This 'normal': muscular activity observed in fluent stutterers under masking would again not support a simple 'distraction' explanation.

However, Venkatagiri (1980) has suggested that genuine and artificial stuttering may share some important features. He examined the recorded DAF-induced dysfluencies of 24 non-stutterers and found that like stutterers, their dysfluency under DAF is characterised by part-word repetitions, high frequency of dysfluency on polysyllabic words, high frequency of dysfluency on initial syllables and adaptation in repeated readings. However, the degree of consistency of stuttering between initial and subsequent oral readings in DAF-induced dysfluency was found to be considerably less. In contrast, Neelly (1961) found that adaptation to repeated oral readings was significantly different in the two groups.

Aphasia, Apraxia and Dysarthria

In recent years there has been increasing interest in the effect of DAF on the speech of aphasic patients. In an early study Stanton (1958) tested thirteen aphasic patients and found that three responded similarly to normal subjects, two were unaffected by the DAF and five benefited. For three other patients, Stanton described responses as 'atypical'. Singh and Schlanger (1969) compared the effects of a DAF delay-time of 180 ms on ten aphasic, ten dysarthric and ten mentally retarded subjects. The aphasic group were described as having mild or moderate 'expressive' aphasia. The aim of the study was to compare sentence duration, vocal intensity and phonemic errors in the three groups during the production of read or repeated sentences of three levels of meaningfulness. The differential performance of the three groups is difficult to assess in this study as the results for the groups are combined in a number of instances. However, sentence durations were distorted in seven aphasic patients, and the level of vocal intensity also increased in the groups as a whole under DAF. Phonemic errors for all groups increased also as a function of the meaningfulness of the sentences with the aphasic group making most errors followed by the dysarthric group and then the mentally retarded group. Moreover, sentence durations were longest, for all three groups taken together, for the least meaningful sentences. Amongst the aphasic subjects, two produced longer sentence durations under the no-delay condition than under DAF and one appeared to be unaffected by DAF. The remaining seven aphasic subjects all experienced some kind of unspecified disruption under DAF. It appears that vocal intensity also increased under DAF for all groups taken together.

The study does not provide sufficient detailed comparison of results for the three groups of subjects and little indication of performance under the no-delay condition. Moreover, there is a minimum of interpretive discussion. However, it would appear to support Stanton's (1958) finding that there is variability in the reaction of aphasic patients to DAF.

A recent series of interesting studies has extended our knowledge of the effects of DAF on aphasic subjects (Vrtunski, Mack, Boller and Kim, 1976; Boller and Marcie, 1978; Boller, Vrtunski, Kim and Mack, 1978; Chapin, Blumstein, Meissner and Boller, 1981) by examining more systematically the role of auditory feedback in aphasia.

Vrtunski *et al*. (1976) compared a left-hemisphere damaged group, a right-hemisphere damaged group and a control group under DAF (360 ms) involving an easy and a difficult verbal task (counting and reporting sentences) and DAF involving an easy and difficult non-verbal task (tapping at a steady rate and tapping a simple Morse Code pattern). The auditory feedback in this non-verbal condition was a 600 Hz tone produced by the tapping pressure. The dependent variables examined were vocal intensity and duration of speech and intensity and duration of tapping.

Of the left-hemisphere damaged group six had Wernicke's, two had Broca's and one had conduction aphasia, and the final subject was not aphasic. All subjects across all groups showed the expected DAF effect on most tasks to some degree.

The interesting finding of this study is that whereas controls showed increased DAF effect on both verbal and non-verbal tasks as the task became more difficult, for the left-hemisphere damaged group with impaired verbal processing the DAF effect reduced as the verbal (but not the non-verbal) task became more difficult. For the right-hemisphere damaged group, however, impaired in non-verbal processing, the DAF effect reduced as the non-verbal (but not the verbal) task became more difficult. The finding that the predominantly aphasic left-hemisphere group all experienced disruption in duration and intensity under DAF is in contrast to the findings of Stanton (1958) and Singh and Schlanger (1969) indicating variability.

Boller *et al.* (1978) explored the effects of DAF at 180 and 360 ms on ten fluent and ten non-fluent aphasic subjects and ten controls. The aim of the study was to measure performance on a number of speech tasks, ranging in difficulty from repetition to answering questions to reading, in terms of the three variables of vocal intensity, duration and articulatory quality of speech. A number of interesting findings emerged in this tightly designed study. First, all subjects across all groups showed some DAF effect and the 180 ms delay was the most effective in causing disturbance on the variables measured. Secondly, fluent aphasic subjects produced a significantly smaller DAF effect than non-fluent subjects and a non-significantly smaller effect than the normal control group. Thirdly, this study failed to find any aphasic subject whose speech improved under DAF, except in reading by the fluent group where speech quality was actually better under DAF than under the no-DAF condition. Even so, duration and intensity were increased for this group and it was articulatory speech quality alone which showed improvements. Furthermore, the smallest DAF effects were produced by three conduction aphasic subjects, who formed a sub-group within the fluent group; and one Broca's subject classified as 'recovered'. Further findings of interest were that there was considerable variability in DAF effect relative to speech task used and that the variable which discriminated best between groups was 'quality of speech'. Correlation analysis suggested to the authors that duration and quality of speech are closely related variables whereas vocal intensity appears to be independent of the other two. This latter suggestion supports Fairbanks' (1955) earlier distinction between 'direct' and 'indirect' effects and the study concludes that an independent monitoring system controls intensity (indirect) which is affected

similarly in aphasic and normal subjects, but a second system responsible for duration and articulatory quality (direct) is affected differently
in different aphasic types.

A follow-up study (Chapin *et al.*, 1981) sought to subject the data
from the Boller *et al.* (1978) study to a detailed examination of the
'speech quality' variable which was shown to be the most discriminating amongst groups. A further aim was to determine which speech
quality errors could be considered phonological and which phonetic
in nature. Phonological errors were processes such as phonemic or
syllabic substitutions, simplifications and additions, and examples of
phonetic errors were increases in length of vowels, fricatives and sonor-
ants. The original aphasic subjects (Boller *et al.*, 1978) were further
subdivided into Broca's, Wernicke's, conduction and posterior (two
word-deaf and one transcortical sensory).

Results of the analysis revealed that the phonetic feature of vowel
length was the only speech quality error which was significantly affected
and none of the phonological measures contributed significantly to
errors in speech quality. Furthermore, the only significant difference
between the groups occurred between conduction subjects who were
the least affected, and Broca's subjects who were the most affected.
The authors conclude firstly, that DAF affects ongoing phonetic
planning and implementation and not phonological processes. They
suggest secondly, that the observation that conduction aphasic patients
are relatively unaffected by DAF supports the *disconnection* explanation of conduction aphasia (Wernicke, 1908; Geschwind, 1965) which
holds that a disconnection between the sensory and motor images
of words underlies this type of aphasia, possibly due to a lesion in the
arcuate fasciculus, the bundle of interconnecting fibres which joins
Wernicke's area and Broca's area. Finally, they interpret the Broca
patients' poor performance under DAF to indicate a highly fragile
articulatory system, supporting the view (Darley *et al.*, 1975; Johns
and LaPointe, 1976; Code and Ball, 1982) that an apraxia of speech
is a significant component of the disorder we call Broca's aphasia. The
findings of a study by Lozano and Dreyer (1978) who investigated
the effects of DAF (180 ms) on the speech of five subjects with fairly
'pure' apraxia of speech supports this general finding. The experimental task involved reading single monosyllabic and polysyllabic
words and the number of speech production errors was calculated.
No significant differences were detected by judges in the number of
errors in the DAF and no-DAF conditions suggested by the researchers
to support the view that apraxia of speech is primarily a motor speech

disorder without auditory system involvement. The problem in interpreting the result of this study is that the use of a single-word reading task rather than longer utterances might have produced the smaller DAF effect. Also, indirect effects were not measured.

The apparently beneficial effect of DAF on the speech of conduction aphasic patients was further examined by Boller and Marcie (1978) who compared a single conduction subject to a group of normal subjects. Subjects were asked to repeat words and a short sentence under no-DAF and DAF (200 ms) and measures used were subjective judgements of intensity, quality and rhythm, a stop-watch measurement of duration and a phonemic analysis of errors. The repetitions of the conduction aphasic patient improved under DAF on all measures whereas the normal subjects showed the expected negative effects of DAF. The authors suggest that this result confirms the view that conduction aphasia entails a delay in what they call 'external phonemic' feedback (at the phonetic actualisation level) as well as a delay in 'internal phonemic' feedback (at the phonological selection level). For normal subjects, DAF interferes only with internal feedback.

In summary, the indicators are that when sufficiently sensitive measures are employed most aphasic subjects show some disturbance in speech production as a result of DAF. It would appear that conduction patients are affected the least (less than normal subjects) and Broca's patients the most. It seems that it is the phonetic aspects of speech quality (mainly vowel length) and duration which are most affected. These variables constitute Fairbanks' indirect effects.

Clinical Applications

Stuttering

The clinical application of DAF in speech pathology has been mainly as a means of training stutterers to reduce their rate of utterance by learning a slower-paced method of speech referred to often as *prolonged speech*. A therapeutic approach which employs DAF as part of an operant treatment programme designed to train prolonged speech, began with work by Goldiamond (1965) and has been developed and described in a number of subsequent studies (Curlee and Perkins, 1969; Ryan, 1971; Ryan and Van Kirk, 1974). The method involves systematic 'step-by-step procedures which include prescribed reinforcement schedules and criterion levels' (Ryan and Van Kirk, 1974: p. 3). The procedures described by Ryan and Van Kirk illustrate well how DAF is used as part of a behavioural programme. The aim of the programme is to establish fluent conversational speech in the clinical setting, to transfer fluency to a variety of settings outside the clinic and finally to maintain fluency over a long period of time. Each of these three phases of the programme (establishment, transfer, maintenance) is made up of a number of steps (in the case of the establishment phase, 27 steps). During the establishment phase the patient is taught first to read, then speak in monologue and finally engage in conversation, in a slow prolonged speech with the aid of DAF. The delay time starts at 250 ms and is gradually reduced in 50 ms steps to a no-delay condition until the patient is using fluent prolonged speech without the aid of DAF. The criterion set for progression to a following step is five minutes of fluency at each step. Ryan and Van Kirk report that the programme, which lasts approximately 20 hours, was effective in establishing and maintaining fluency in a large population of stutterers of both sexes with a wide range of ages and varying degrees of severity.

Van Riper (1970, 1973) has proposed a number of therapeutic applications of DAF with stutterers based on clinical observation. He suggests that at an early stage of therapy the clinician can demonstrate the effects of DAF on his or her own speech and thereby show the patient that normal speakers can be made to stutter. DAF can also be used to show the patient that stuttered speech is modifiable. Van Riper also advocates a procedure which trains the patient to ignore auditory feedback and rely instead on proprioceptive and tactile feedback. Through a systematic behavioural approach the stutterer learns to 'beat the machine', as Van Riper puts it, and becomes more fluent through reliance on forms of feedback other than auditory.

With the recent silicone chip revolution, body-worn DAF devices like those described in an earlier section, will hopefully become cheaper and more accessible. Body-worn devices may then be used to a much greater extent in the stutterers everyday life. This should improve control over the transfer and maintenance stages of a therapeutic programme. Low and Lindsay (1979) suggest that ultimately a 'behind-the-ear' device will be produced. With the current growth in miniaturisation, such an aid should not be far away. These developments are to be welcomed. Low and Lindsay state, however, that there is a degree of consumer resistance to such devices and milder stutterers were not greatly helped by the constantly available DAF. Moreover, although no details of trials were given, they suggest that the improvement observed in severe stutterers reduces with time. It is clear that properly designed studies are required to determine the clinical value of this technological development.

Applications with Other Communication Disorders

There are indications from a recent report (Downie, Low and Lindsay, 1981) that DAF may have a therapeutic application in the management of Parkinson's disease. This trial examined the responses of eleven hyperkinetic dysarthria patients suffering from Parkinson's disease to the body-worn Aberdeen Speech Aid. Of the eleven patients who tried the device two showed dramatic improvements in their speech, one showed slight improvement and the rest did not benefit. Of the two patients who benefited from DAF, one whose speech without DAF was characterised by hesitations, repetitions, excessive rate and short rushes of words, showed dramatic improvement under a delay time of 50 ms (but not 200 ms). The DAF was of great benefit for three months, but original speech patterns began to return after this and after twelve months the DAF was discontinued. The other patient who benefited had speech which was low in intensity and excessive in rate, a classical Parkinsonian dysarthria. The patient had had some kind of stutter in early life which he felt had returned since the development of Parkinson's disease. After two years using the DAF device at 50 ms delay time, his speech remains totally fluent with a reduced rate and an improvement in intensity. Those Parkinson patients who did not benefit had either mild speech problems or showed marked akinetic features and slow faint speech. The authors conclude that Parkinson's patients with festinant speech may benefit from permanently available DAF. Properly organised therapy programmes, supervised by speech pathologists, may hold promise for such patients and trials might also examine the therapeutic applications of DAF for other types of dysarthria.

From the above review of DAF investigation in aphasia, it seems that there are indications that DAF has a beneficial effect on the speech quality of conduction aphasic patients and Wernicke's patients while reading, although no major therapeutic application of DAF with such patients has been exploited. It would appear that Broca's aphasics, and others with apraxia of speech, do not benefit from DAF. There may, however, be a *clinical* contribution of DAF to be exploited, in aiding diagnosis and prognosis. It may be, for instance, that DAF could be used to help determine the integrity of the auditory-motor speech system in fluent patients and the fragility of articulatory planning in non-fluent patients (Chapin *et al.*, 1981). Code (1982) has suggested that DAF could be useful in assessing the self-monitoring capabilities of patients with recurrent utterance, as an improvement in self-monitoring usually precedes the break-up of the recurrent utterance and the emergence of agrammatic speech. DAF might also prove useful as part of a therapeutic programme to improve the self-monitoring abilities of various types of aphasic patients.

Conclusion

DAF is a technique which has had wide application in speech science since its effects were first described over thirty years ago. It has contributed to knowledge concerning the role of auditory feedback in the control of ongoing speech production in normal subjects and has shed light on the development of auditory feedback from childhood to adulthood. It has also had a significant impact on theoretical explanations of stuttering, and has been successfully applied to therapeutic management. Recent work indicates that carefully designed studies, employing a range of tasks and clearly identified measures of change, can contribute to our understanding of neurological and neuropsychological disorders of communication which may provide future help in clinical management, and the recent development of a number of body-worn DAF devices will enable the application of DAF beyond the clinic.

8 TIME-VARIATED SPEECH

Linda L. Riensche, Daniel J. Orchik and
Daniel S. Beasley

Introduction

Research and application of time-varied speech signals is confined
predominantly to the past 25 years, with those investigations of direct
pertinence to speech-language pathology and audiology occurring
primarily within the past decade. In this chapter, a general description
of the several techniques for modifying the temporal characteristics
of the speech signal will be presented, followed by a discussion of
some research with normal and disordered adults and children relative to the intelligibility and comprehension of time-altered speech.

Procedures for Temporally Distorting Speech

Beasley and Maki (1976) have described in detail several methods of
time-varying speech stimuli, including alteration in speaking rate
and recorded playback speed as well as manual, electromechanical
and computerised sampling procedures. Speaking rate variation simply
entails speaking at a different rate. While this is a convenient method,
it is limited to the range of human speaking rates available and also in
the reliability of the resulting speech signals. That is, most individuals
can only increase their rates by about 30 per cent and have difficulty
controlling the overall duration of the signal, vocal inflections, con-
sonant-vowel and pause durations, and coarticulatory interactions.
Playback rate variation entails playing a recorded message at a rate
different from the rate at which it was originally recorded. This method
also is simple and convenient, but it introduces artifacts into the resultant signal in the form of frequency shifts which are proportional to
the resultant time shift.

Sampling procedures entail modifications of a recorded signal by
discarding and retaining portions of the signal, thereby minimising
the distorting effects of frequency alteration. Manual sampling requires
removal of portions of the recorded material and then splicing together

the remaining portions of the recorded signal. This method allows for selection of those portions to be discarded and retained and provides for the addition of silent intervals of selected duration, but the procedure is time consuming and tedious.

Electromechanical sampling entails the use of an electromechanical time compressor/expander, first developed by Fairbanks, Everitt and Jaeger (1954). The Fairbanks device allows for the recording of a signal and then, through the use of a tape loop, temporally compressing the signal by deleting portions of it during the playback process, and simultaneously abutting the remaining portions. Temporal expansion of a signal can be accomplished by insertion of repeated samples during the playback process. This method is convenient but does not allow selection of specific portions to be discarded or retained, and the required technology is bulky and expensive.

Electronic sampling entails the use of an electronic time compressor/expander, such as the Lexicon Varispeech developed by Lee (1972). Lee's device employs the principles of the electromechanical time compressor/expander through the use of a minicomputer and tape recorder. The Lexicon is portable, inexpensive, and exemplifies the current state of the art for applied research of time-variated speech. In the future, however, mini- and microcomputers will most likely become increasingly useful in both research and clinical application.

Intelligibility

Investigations of the intelligibility of time-variated speech have included the use of various stimulus materials such as words, phrases and sentences, variations in signal characteristics such as interstimulus intervals, and a variety of populations. For normal-hearing listeners, speech which has been time-varied using a playback rate variation technique has been found to be significantly less intelligible than that employing sampling procedures (Garvey, 1953; Klumpp and Webster, 1961; McLain, 1962; Fletcher, 1965; Foulke, 1966; Daniloff, Shriner and Zemlin, 1968). With both methods, intelligibility decreases with decreasing signal duration, with dramatic reductions in intelligibility occurring at about a 33 per cent decrease in duration (33 per cent time compression) for the playback rate variation technique and at about a 70 per cent decrease in duration (70 per cent time compression) for the sampling methods. Other factors found to affect the intelligibility of normal listeners are the size of the discard interval (Fairbanks and Kodman, 1957) and linguistic complexity of the stimuli (Klumpp and Webster, 1961).

Time-compressed speech stimuli have been assumed to have potential for assessment of lesions in the auditory cortex, based upon the results of clinical studies which used distorted signals with patients presenting such lesions (Bordley and Haskins, 1955; Calearo, Teatini and Pestalozza, 1962; Katz, 1962; Jerger, 1964; Speaks and Jerger, 1965). Subsequent research suggesting that the auditory perceptual system was temporally biased (Hirsh, 1967; Aaronson, 1967; Beasley and Shriner, 1973) lent support to these earlier contentions. Calearo and Lazzaroni (1957) discussed the rationale for use of time-compressed speech stimuli for clinical purposes in terms of the role played by external and internal redundancy in speech perception. External redundancy refers to the redundancy inherent in the speech signal. That is, the acoustic and linguistic characteristics of speech, together with the interactions between their respective components, provide significantly more information than necessary to permit normal processing of speech signals to take place. Internal redundancy, on the other hand, refers to the neurophysiological redundancy of the central auditory system *per se*, as evidenced by the many contralateral and ipsilateral neural pathways and interconnections known to be present in the central nervous system. The inherent redundancy within the human nervous system permits normal performance on traditional speech discrimination tests, even if a portion of the nervous system is damaged. If the external temporal redundancy is reduced, for example through the process of time compression, the internal redundancy of the normal auditory system could be expected to compensate for the reduced temporal nature of the signal, resulting in normal intelligibility. If the central auditory system suffers neural pathology, however, then compensation for signal distortion would be reduced.

Adults

Normal Populations

In recent years, there have been efforts to develop standardised procedures and normative data for time-altered speech signals in order to overcome earlier equivocal findings with clinical populations. This has lead, in turn, to more systematic study of time-altered speech with persons presenting disorders of communication. Beasley, Schwimmer and Rintelmann (1972b) suggested that some of the earlier investigations of time-altered speech which demonstrated equivocal results may have suffered from experimental design problems and methodological difficulties, including small population sample sizes and inappropriately easy test stimuli as well as low percentages of time compression and inappropriately high levels of presentation. Others failed to provide adequate normative data and to use standard procedures for time compressing the stimuli, a criticism which has been noted as a major problem with many measures of auditory processing (Beasley and Freeman, 1977; Willeford, 1976).

Consequently, in a series of three investigations, Beasley and his associates obtained normative data on the performance of young normal-hearing adults who were presented time-compressed mono-syllabic stimuli. Beasley *et al.* (1972b) obtained normative data on the performance of 96 normal-hearing young adults who were presented four monosyllabic word lists at 0 per cent (normal), 30, 40, 50, 60 and 70 per cent time compression at sensation levels of 8, 16, 24, and 32 db, respectively. The word lists used by Beasley *et al.* (1972b) were the Rintelmann and Jetty (1968) recorded versions of Form B and the Northwestern University Auditory Test No. 6 (NU-6) (Tillman and Carhart, 1966). The words in each list were time-compressed via an electromechanical time-compressor/expander calibrated according to the procedures described by Konkle *et al.* (1977b). Results of this study, shown in Figure 8.1, indicated that intelligibility increased with increased sensation level but gradually decreased with increasing percentage of time compression, to 60 per cent, followed by a dramatic breakdown in intelligibility at 70 per cent time compression. These data were expanded to include a 40 dB sensation level by Beasley, Forman and Rintelmann (1972a), who presented the same stimuli to another group of normal-hearing young adults and obtained a slight but non-significant improvement in scores over those obtained by Beasley *et al.* (1972b) at 32 dB sensation level (see Table 8.1). In a related investigation, Riensche, Konkle and Beasley (1976), using 80 normal-hearing young adults, found that results of time-compressed versions of Form A of the NU-6 replicated the trends in the earlier study by Beasley *et al.* (1972b).

The normative data for time-compressed monosyllabic stimuli also have been extended to geriatric populations. Konkle, Beasley and Bess (1977a) presented the Beasley *et al.* (1972a, b) NU-6 word lists to 118 persons divided into four age groups (54 to 60 years; 61 to 67 years; 68 to 74 years; and 75 years and older). The words were time-compressed by 0, 20, 40 and 60 per cent and presented at sensation levels of 24, 32, and 40 dB. The subjects had hearing thresholds typical for their age and good discrimination abilities when presented

Figure 8.1: Mean Percentage Correct Scores for Normal-hearing Young Adult Listeners on the Four NU-6 Monosyllabic Word Lists, under Time Compression Conditions of 0 per cent and 30 to 70 per cent in 10 per cent Steps, each List and Compression Condition Presented at Each of Four Sensation Levels (8, 16, 24, 32 dB)

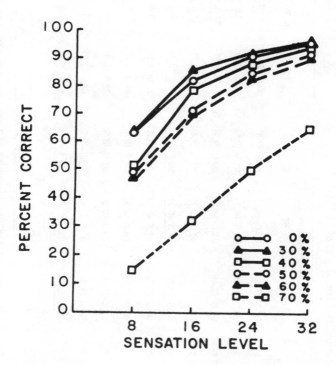

Source: Reprinted with permission from Beasley *et al.* (1972b).

with traditional discrimination tests. Results (Figure 8.2) demonstrated improved performance with increased sensation level and decreased percentage of time compression, but performance as reflected in the mean scores was distinctly poorer than that for young adults and became increasingly poorer with increasing age. These results have been confirmed in subsequent studies by Echols-Chambers (1981) and Clasquin (1980).

Table 8.1: Mean Percent Correct Scores and Standard Deviations (in parenthesis) for Normal Hearing Young Adults for Each of Four Lists of the NU-6 Monosyllabic Words, each time-compressed by 0% (normal) and 30% through 70% in 10 steps, and presented at 32 dB sensation level (Beasley et al., 1972a)

	0	30	40	Time-Compression (%) 50	60	70	M̄ TOTAL
SL LIST							
32 I	95.5 (3.2)	98.0 (1.6)	92.5 (1.9)	90.0 (4.9)	85.5 (3.4)	60.0 (7.5)	86.9(13.5)
II	97.0 (1.2)	95.5 (3.4)	93.5 (3.8)	95.5 (4.1)	91.5 (2.5)	64.0 (3.3)	89.5(12.1)
III	95.5 (1.0)	94.0 (1.6)	91.5 (3.4)	91.0 (4.2)	92.0 (3.3)	64.0(10.7)	88.0(12.0)
IV	97.5 (1.1)	99.0 (1.2)	98.5 (1.0)	93.0 (7.7)	92.5 (4.4)	74.0 (4.3)	92.4 (9.5)
M̄ TOTAL	96.3 (2.0)	96.6 (2.8)	94.0 (3.7)	92.3 (5.3)	90.3 (4.3)	65.5 (8.3)	89.2
40 I	99.5 (1.0)	97.0 (2.0)	97.0 (3.8)	93.5 (3.4)	95.5 (2.5)	72.0(15.0)	92.4(11.2)
II	97.0 (3.5)	97.0 (3.5)	97.0 (3.5)	98.0 (2.3)	89.5 (6.6)	84.0 (3.6)	93.8 (6.4)
III	97.5 (3.0)	95.0 (1.6)	96.0 (1.6)	93.0 (3.5)	96.0 (3.6)	79.0 (2.6)	92.9 (6.3)
IV	98.5 (1.9)	99.5 (1.0)	98.5 (1.9)	97.5 (1.9)	95.5 (2.5)	86.5 (3.0)	96.0 (4.9)
M̄ TOTAL	98.1 (2.5)	97.4 (2.4)	97.1 (2.7)	95.5 (3.5)	94.1 (4.7)	80.4 (9.1)	93.8
M̄ SL Difference	1.8	0.8	3.1	3.2	3.8	14.9	4.6

Source: Reprinted with permission from D. Beasley et al. (1972a). Perception of time-compressed CNC monosyllables by normal listeners. *Journal of Auditory Research, 12,* 71-5.

Figure 8.2: Mean Percentage Correct Scores for Adults in Four Age Groups Compared to a Group of Young Adults (Beasley *et al*, 1972b) in Response to Presentation of Time-Compressed (0 per cent, 20 per cent, 40 per cent, 60 per cent) Versions of the NU-6 Word Lists at Three Sensation Level Conditions (24, 32 and 40 dB)

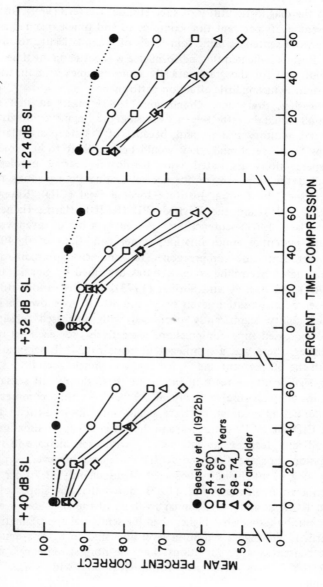

Source: Reprinted with permission from Konkle *et al.* (1977a).

Several investigators have studied the effects of grammaticalness, stimulus length, and presentation rate on the perception of sentential stimuli, (that is, sentences or approximations to normal sentences as described by Miller, 1956), thereby providing the impetus for research into the diagnostic utility of such stimuli. Gerver (1969), for example, presented 50 per cent time-compressed and time-expanded seven- and nine-word sentences using four levels of grammaticality to adult listeners. Results indicated that performance was better on the time-expanded stimuli and for the grammatically more complex stimuli, with length apparently having little effect on performance.

Beasley, Bratt and Rintelmann (1980) suggested that sentential stimuli could be effective in assessing the linguistic integrity of the central auditory system, and, because of the steep articulation functions for these stimuli, they would be less likely to be subject to the misperceptions associated with peripheral hearing problems. They studied the responses of 96 normal-hearing young adults to presentations of the Central Institute for the Deaf (CID) (Silverman and Hirsh, 1955) and the Revised CID (RCID) (Harris, Haines, Kelsey and Clark, 1961) sentence lists as well as a list of seven-word, third-order sentential approximations under conditions of 0, 40, 60 and 70 per cent time compression. The sentential approximations were constructed according to procedures described by Speaks and Jerger (1965) and Beasley and Shriner (1973), and the various stimuli were presented at sensation levels of 24 and 40 dB. As shown in Table 8.2, intelligibility significantly decreased with decreased sensation level and increased time compression, respectively, for each set of stimuli. Further, there was a significant decrease of 24 dB sensation level in both the 60 per cent and 70 per cent compression conditions, whereas, the significant decrease in intelligibility at the 40 dB sensation level condition was observed only at 70 per cent time compression. The sentential approximations were significantly more difficult than were the CID and RCID sentences, and the sentential approximations showed significant decreases in intelligibilty with each increase in time compression. For the CID and RCID sentences, however, a precipitous decrease in intelligibility occurred predominantly at 70 per cent time compression. Beasley *et al.* (1980) noted that the slopes of the CID and RCID stimuli were similar to those of the time-compressed NU-6 stimuli, but somewhat higher than the sentential approximation scores. Further, the higher sensation level appeared to be less beneficial for the sentential approximations than the normal sentences, underscoring the distinct advantages for intelligibility with normal linguistic stimuli.

Table 8.2: Mean Percent Correct Scores for Normal Hearing Young Adults for Two Lists of Normal Sentences (CID and RCID) and One List of 2nd Order Sentential Approximations, each sentence time-compressed by 0% (normal) and 40% through 70% in 10% steps and presented at 24 dB and 40 dB sensation levels

Test	SL	Time Compression (%)				Grand Mean
		0	40	60	70	
CID	24	99.4	99.2	97.5	70.4	91.6
	40	99.6	98.9	97.9	82.1	94.6
	Mean	99.5	99.0	97.7	76.2	93.1
RICD	24	99.7	99.4	97.7	71.0	91.9
	40	99.4	99.2	98.3	83.3	95.0
	Mean	99.6	99.3	97.5	77.1	93.5
SA	24	96.9	94.0	84.9	42.7	79.6
	40	98.3	94.1	91.4	51.3	83.8
	Mean	97.6	94.1	88.1	47.0	81.7
Grand Mean	24	98.9	97.5	94.6	66.8	89.4
	40	98.7	97.5	93.4	61.4	87.8
		99.1	97.4	95.9	72.3	91.2

Source: Reprinted with permission from D. Beasley *et al.* (1980). Intelligibility of time-compressed sentential stimuli. *Journal of Speech and Hearing Research, 23,* 722-31.

Riensche and Slate (1981) presented the Beasley *et al.* (1980) sentences at 0, 40 and 60 per cent compression ratios to three groups of teenagers (12.5 to 13.5 years; 14.5 to 15.5 years; and 16.5 to 17.5 years of age) at 45 and 60 dB SPL. They chose to present the stimuli at SPL (Sound Pressure Level) levels because of the greater convenience for use in public school testing and because of the inaccuracies potentially introduced when attempting to find very low speech reception threshold (SRT) levels. Findings indicated a slight improvement in performance with increased age, but were essentially in agreement with results obtained from adults at the 24 and 40 dB sensation levels.

Freeman and Church (1977) extended the data on time-compressed sentential stimuli by presenting four lists of five-word first-order sentential approximations to 40 normal-hearing young adults at sensation levels of 16, 24, 32, and 40 dB. The lists were presented at each of four time compression ratios: 0, 20, 40 and 60 per cent. Increased sensation level reflected improved performance only on the 60 per cent time-compressed condition, the compression level which showed the major detrimental effect on auditory discrimination performance.

Finally, the effect of word list and talker variation on time-compressed speech discrimination scores were highlighted by De Chicchis, Orchik and Tecca (1981). The Central Institute for the Deaf (CID) W-22 (Hirsh *et al.*, 1952) and NU-6 word lists were studied using commercially available recordings (Auditec of St Louis). Also the performance on the Auditec NU-6 recordings were compared to the data from the original recordings by Beasley *et al.* (1972b), who used a different talker for the NU-6. Results indicated that different word lists with ostensibly similar difficulty levels under normal conditions may, in fact, give dissimilar results when altered in some ways, as in temporal distortions. Further, the effect of talker variation was even more dramatic, in that scores for the Auditec recordings of the NU-6 were markedly poorer at all levels of time compression than those obtained for the Beasley recordings.

Clinical Populations

Although early investigators of the use of time-varied speech with clinical populations obtained equivocal findings (Calearo and Lazzaroni, 1957; Bocca and Calearo, 1963; de Quiros, 1964; Luterman, Welsh and Melrose, 1966; Sticht and Gray, 1969), they nevertheless stimulated interest in the clinical use of such stimuli. Recently, a number of investigators have employed the time-compressed versions of the NU-6 and other stimuli to investigate the auditory perceptual abilities of adult clinical populations. Their findings suggest that these stimuli may be effective in detecting diffuse lesions of the temporal lobe, but that the information they provide should be interpreted with the findings obtained from other measures (Echols-Chambers, (1981). That is, they should be employed as part of a battery of tests (Beasley and Freeman, 1977; Willeford, 1976).

Kurdziel, Noffsinger and Olsen (1976) presented the time-compressed NU-6 stimuli to 16 subjects having surgically induced discrete right or left temporal lobe lesions and 15 subjects having diffuse unilateral cortical lesions involving at least the temporal lobe. The performance of the subjects having discrete anterior temporal lobe lesions showed little difference between ears or percentages of time compression. However, the performance of the subjects having diffuse temporal lobe lesions was characterised by poorer performance in the ear contralateral to the lesion compared to the ear ipsilateral to the lesion. Also a greater difference between the scores at 0 per cent and 60 per cent time compression was observed for the ear contralateral to the lesion than for the ipsilateral ear.

In another investigation involving brain-damaged adults, Snow, Rintelmann, Miller and Konkle (1977) demonstrated the usefulness of the time-compressed version of the NU-6 in conjunction with the Synthetic Sentence Identification (SSI) test (Jerger, 1970). They presented the SSI and the time-compressed NU-6 stimuli to a 42-year-old woman who had suffered a cerebro-vascular accident involving the left temporal lobe. Results of the SSI suggested brainstem involvement, but performance on the time-compressed stimuli indicated temporal lobe dysfunction as well, a finding which was later confirmed.

In an investigation employing eight adult aphasic subjects and a matched control group, Orchik, Walker and Larson (1977) found that the aphasic subject group performed poorer than the control group at all levels on the Word Intelligibility by Picture Identification test (WIPI) (Ross and Lerman, 1970), presented under 0, 30 and 60 per cent time-compression conditions. The greatest difference in performance was at 60 per cent time compression. Further, the aphasic subjects demonstrated comparable performance to that of their control subjects at 0 and 30 per cent time compression in at least one ear, thereby suggesting that the WIPI may be a more appropriate measure for use with aphasic patients than the conventional open set speech discrimination measures typically used with adults. In addition, though two subjects demonstrated suppressed performance in the ear contralateral to what appeared to be the damaged hemisphere, one subject demonstrated suppressed performance in the ear ipsilateral to what appeared to be the damaged hemisphere, lending further support to the argument for using a battery of tests in assessing central auditory processing function.

The performance of subjects presenting peripheral hearing losses also has been reported for time-compressed stimuli. Kurdziel, Rintelmann and Beasley (1975) examined the performance of nine men having noise-induced sensorineural hearing losses. Articulation functions of the group were similar to those obtained for normal-hearing subjects, but mean scores were lower than normal at each time-compression condition. At 0 per cent and 30 per cent time compression, PB—MAX occurred at 32 and 24 dB sensation level, respectively, rather than at 40 dB sensation level. The investigators suggested that when using time-compressed stimuli with this type of population, an optimum intelligibility score needs to be obtained. Also the differences between scores at 0 and 40 per cent time compression for peripheral-hearing loss subjects can be expected to range from 10 per cent to 15 per cent or higher, compared to less than 3 per cent for normal-hearing subjects.

Another investigation employing the time-compressed stimuli was designed to examine peripheral and central auditory function among patients having sickle cell anaemia. Sharp and Orchik (1978) noted that the diffuse effects of sickle cell crisis might be expected to produce both peripheral and central auditory dysfunction. They presented time-compressed NU-6 and WIPI stimuli to nine subjects having sickle cell anaemia and to a matched control group. Measures of peripheral hearing abilities indicated no evidence of impairment. However, scores on the time-compressed stimuli were on the average about 5 to 15 per cent poorer in the left and right ears, respectively, for the sickle cell subjects compared to the control group, thereby indicating reduced central auditory function. It was suggested that further research is needed to determine correlations between central auditory skills and the number, duration, and severity of sickle cell crisis episodes as well as to examine the influence of other haemolytic disorders on central auditory function.

Time-compressed sentences have been employed in the assessment of the auditory perceptual abilities of adults. Doran and Riensche (1981) presented the 0, 40 and 60 per cent time-compressed CID, RCID, and sentential approximations used by Beasley *et al.* (1980) to a group of stuttering and non-stuttering adult subjects at sensation levels of 24 and 32 dB. The performance levels of the two groups were

Figure 8.3: Mean Percentage Correct Scores for Normal-hearing Children in Three Age Groups (4, 6 and 8 years) on Presentations of Time-compressed (0, 30 and 60 per cent) Versions of the PB-K 50 (a) and WIPI (b) Word Lists, Each Presented at Two Sensation Levels (16 and 32dB)

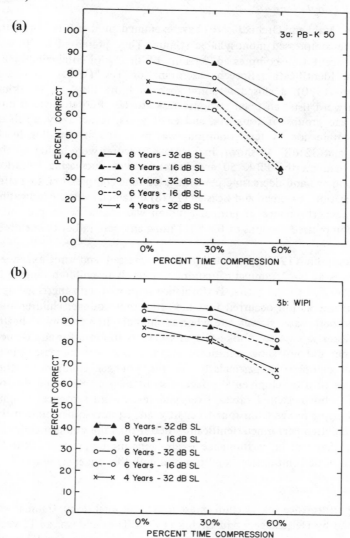

Source: Reprinted with permission from Beasley *et al.* (1976).

similar though there was a subtle difference in the pattern of performance over the various time-compression levels.

Children

Normal Populations

Beasley, Maki and Orchik (1976) have examined children's performance
on time-compressed monosyllabic stimuli. They presented 0, 30, and
60 per cent time-compressed versions of the Word Intelligibility by
Picture Identification Speech Discrimination Test (WIPI) (Ross and
Lerman, 1970), a closed response task, and the PB-K 50 (Haskins,
1949) word lists, an open response task, to 60 children divided into
three age groups of four, six, and eight years, respectively. Each of
the compression by test conditions was presented at sensation levels
of 16 and 32 dB. As shown in Figure 8.3, scores were higher on the
WIPI than on the PB-K 50 and increased with increasing sensation
level and age and decreasing percentage of time compression. In a later
investigation, Freeman and Beasley (1978) obtained evidence indicating
that the performance of normal children was similar when presented
time-compressed versions of the WIPI using an open, rather than closed,
format.

Thompson (1973) presented time-compressed and time-expanded
sentences at two grammatical complexity levels to children ranging in
age from 5.6 to 9.6 years. Performance improved with increased age,
but an interaction occurred that indicated that younger children performed better at a slower rate whereas older children performed better
at a faster rate. Also, unlike Gerver's (1969) findings for adults, performance did not show significant improvement with increased grammatical complexity, particularly for the younger children. Further
evidence of a developmental effect was obtained by King and Weston
(1974) who presented three-, five-, and seven-word sentences to children ranging in age from four to eight years. Results indicated that the
older children performed significantly better than the younger children,
with differences in performance levels being more apparent at the 50
per cent time compression condition and with the longer sentences.

Clinical Populations

The performance of a child presenting temporal lobe trauma was
reported by Oelschlaeger and Orchik (1977). The child was an 11-year-
old girl with confirmed left hemisphere damage and normal hearing
as evidenced by pure tone thresholds and impedance testing. At 0 per

cent time compression, she obtained scores of 96 per cent and 88 per cent in the left and right ears, respectively. However, under 60 per cent time compression, she obtained scores of 68 per cent and 32 per cent for the left and right ears, respectively, a trend which was reported in earlier research with brain-damaged adults (Kurdziel *et al.*, 1976). That is, performance was poorer in the ear contralateral to the lesion and the difference score between 0 and 60 per cent time compression was greater for the ear contralateral to the lesion.

Several investigators also have used the time-compressed monosyllabic stimuli to examine the performance of children having learning and articulatory production problems. Manning, Johnston and Beasley (1977) presented the time-compressed version of the PB-K 50 stimuli to 20 children diagnosed as having auditory perceptual disorders. The subjects performed equally well at the 0 per cent and 30 per cent time-compression levels but significantly poorer at 60 per cent time compression. That is, performance by the disordered children was similar to normal children at 30 per cent time compression, but poorer than normal under both the 0 per cent and 60 per cent time-compression conditions.

The time-compressed WIPI stimuli have been studied with children having reading and articulatory production problems (Orchik and Oelschlaeger, 1977; Ormson and Williams, 1975; Orchik, Holgate and Danko, 1979; Freeman and Beasley, 1978). Beasley and Freeman (1977) noted that the results of the several investigations to date had shown different group mean scores under a variety of time-compression conditions, but the difference scores between the 0 per cent and 60 per cent conditions were similar between studies and greater than those for normal-hearing children. They suggested that any child having a difference score greater than 10 per cent on the time-compressed version of the WIPI presented in a closed set format at 24 dB or greater sensation level should be followed closely for auditory perceptual problems. Support for this contention comes from an investigation of the performance of children having mild, moderate, or severe bilateral sensorineural hearing losses without known auditory learning problems. Maki, Beasley, Shoup and Bess (1976) found that the absolute performance of these children on the time-compressed WIPI was significantly affected by the degree of hearing loss, but, regardless of degree of loss, difference scores between 0 per cent and 60 per cent time compression consistently ranged between 10 and 15 per cent.

Freeman and Beasley (1978) used time-compressed versions of three- and five-word first- and second-order sentential approximations and normal sentences (Beasley and Flaherty-Rintelmann, 1976), as well as the time-compressed WIPI stimuli, to examine the performance of reading-impaired and normal-reading children. The reading-impaired children made more errors than the normal-reading children at all percentages of time compression, measured for each of three error types (omissions, substitutions, and additions). Further, the data supported Freeman's (1977) suggestion that 0 per cent and 40 per cent time-compressed sentential approximations could be used effectively as a clinical tool with children.

Riensche and Clauser (1982) employed the 0 per cent and 60 per cent time-compressed 5-word first- and second-order sentential approximations and normal sentences to examine the performance of normal children with a history of severe misarticulation problems, compared to that of a control group of children having no history of age-inappropriate misarticulations. They found that the children having the history of severe misarticulation problems performed significantly poorer than those having no history of such problems. In addition, parents' responses to the questions on the Fisher Auditory Problems Checklist (Fisher, 1980) yielded mean scores of 75 per cent for children with histories of disorders of articulation and 94 per cent for children without such histories. Parents of the formerly misarticulating children more frequently expressed concerns that their children did not listen carefully to directions, were distracted by background sounds and were, or had been, below average in academic areas such as spelling or reading. Riensche and Clauser (1982) recommended that children who receive articulation therapy should be examined for auditory perceptual problems before being dismissed from therapy.

Research investigators have provided an array of information necessary for the interpretation of findings obtained using the time-compressed monosyllabic and sentential stimuli. As suggested earlier, however, the use of time-compressed stimuli in tracking the nature of certain pathological conditions, such as crises episodes in sickle cell anaemia and other haemolytic blood disorders, needs further investigation. Further, preliminary research suggests that subtle ear differences as a function of cerebral dominance occasionally may exist, though confirmation of such an effect has been elusive (Van Ort, Beasley and Riensche, 1979; Riensche and Beasley, 1979; Patterson and Riensche, 1979).

Comprehension

Foulke (1971) has presented an extensive discussion pertaining to the comprehension of time-compressed speech which indicates that the comprehension of speech decreases dramatically beyond 50 per cent time compression. Beasley and Maki (1976) argued that these findings implied that the major detrimental effects of time compression were associated with stimulus intelligibility. In a related study, Sticht (1969) found that time-compressed speech had a more adverse effect on subjects with high mental aptitude than on subjects with low mental aptitude. It was noted, however, that the subjects with low mental aptitude also did more poorly on a discrimination task, suggesting that the primary problem may have been one of intelligibility rather than comprehension. Sticht also reported that the addition of linguistic cues such as prosodic characteristics seem to contribute to improved performance, but contrary to previously reported results (Fairbanks, Guttman and Miron, 1957), simple repetition of the time-compressed passages did not contribute to an improvement in performance.

Other investigators have examined the potential of time-expanded speech as a means to improve listeners' perceptual judgements of speech productions. Using an electromechanical technique, Lass and Foulke (1976) presented 0 per cent, 150 per cent and 200 per cent time-expanded speech samples from misarticulating speakers to 36 student clinicians in training and found that a significantly greater number of misarticulations were identified accurately with increased time expansion. Manning, Lee and Lass (1978) presented 0 per cent, 150 per cent and 200 per cent time-expanded speech samples of stutterers to 30 graduate student clinicians for identification of the occurrence of one-, two- and three-unit part-word repetitions. Significantly more accurate identifications of one-unit part-word repetitions occurred under the 150 per cent and 200 per cent time-expanded conditions compared to normal recordings, though no improvement occurred in the identification of two- and three-unit part-word repetitions. Leeper *et al.* (1980) examined the potential value of time-expanded speech as an aid in improving listeners' perceptual judgements of hypernasality in connected speech samples. They presented 25 samples of various degrees of hypernasal speech time-expanded by 0 per cent, 125 per cent and 175 per cent to inexperienced and experienced student clinicians for ratings of degree of hypernasality and associated confidence measures of each rating. Findings indicated that the listeners' confidence in their judgements increased and the variability of their judgements decreased under the time-expanded conditions.

Clinical investigators have attempted to facilitate comprehension by aphasic persons through the presentation of time-varied speech stimuli. The rationale for the use of such stimuli with this population is based on evidence that the aphasic deficit is at least partially temporal in nature (Efron, 1963; Ebbin and Edwards, 1967; Carpenter and Rutherford, 1973; Cermak and Moreines, 1976; Tallal and Newcombe, 1978). Using slowed speech, Albert and Bear (1974) and Gardner, Albert and Weintraub (1975) reported improvement in the comprehension performance of aphasic subjects, although other investigators have obtained conflicting results.

Brookshire (1973) suggested that some individuals may be unable to receive and process information at the same time and would, therefore, benefit from the strategic insertion of pauses within the speech signal. Liles and Brookshire (1975), using the Token Test, found that the performance of 20 aphasic subjects showed improvement under a five-second pause condition compared to the standard (no pause) condition, with the pause location having no substantial effect on performance. Sheehan, Aseltine and Edwards (1973) examined the comprehension of 30 aphasic subjects under conditions including normal production, interpolated silence around each phoneme, and interword pauses and found that aphasics under 50 years of age showed improved performance only under the interpolated silence condition. Older aphasics, on the other hand, were not significantly affected by either pause condition. In contrast, when Salvatore and Brookshire (1978) attempted to verify the findings by examining the performance of 10 aphasic and 10 non-aphasic subjects, they found that regardless of age, both aphasic and non-aphasic subjects performed less well under interpolated silence conditions than under either of the other conditions. When Salvatore (1975) examined the effects of pause duration, he obtained evidence that a pause of at least two seconds was associated with significant improvement on Token Test commands. Further, subjects exposed to commands characterised by inserted pauses over a four-day training period performed significantly better than subjects who had not received such training.

Electromechanical time-alteration techniques have also been used to study comprehension with aphasic patients. Gordon (1970) presented electromechanically time-expanded Token Test commands to aphasic, non-aphasic brain-damaged, and normal subjects and found that only the aphasic group demonstrated improved, though not statistically significant, performance. Weidner and Lasky (1976) found that aphasic subjects demonstrated significantly improved performance on selected subtests of the Minnesota Test for Differential Diagnosis of Aphasia when the stimuli were time expanded. Lasky, Weidner, and Johnson (1976) combined electronic time-expansion and pause-insertion techniques to alter sentences and found that comprehension significantly improved under both the time-expansion and pause-insertion conditions, but was most effective with the combination of the two forms of distortion.

Findings of other investigators indicate that improved comprehension with time-expanded speech signals may be subject selective, a contention supported by findings that auditory comprehension impairment in aphasia shows a variety of patterns (Brookshire, 1973). Parkhurst (1970) presented time-compressed and time-expanded Token Test commands to aphasic subjects and found that scores decreased under time compression but improved under time expansion for some subjects, particularly when the subjects were given commands. In a similar investigation, Blanchard and Prescott (1980) presented normal and time-expanded versions of the Revised Token Test to 23 aphasic subjects and found improved performance with increased time expansion for 15 of the subjects. Riensche, Wohlert and Porch (1980) reasoned that aphasics may prefer to listen to a rate that facilitates their comprehension. They examined subject's preferred listening rates relative to their comprehension of normal and time-expanded Revised Token Test commands, but failed to obtain definitive evidence of the aphasics' preference ratings relative to the facilitation of comprehension. Examination of subjects' preferred rates relative to their case histories and comprehension abilities yielded a significant correlation only between their preferred rate and number of years of education, whereby subjects having fewer years of education preferred slower rates.

The findings reported in these numerous investigations of comprehension of temporally distorted speech by aphasic patients, though equivocal, cannot be ignored and indicate a need for a better understanding of the temporal nature of the aphasic deficit as well as the application of time-varied stimuli to the diagnostic and therapeutic processes with these patients. For example, the clinician's presentation of test stimuli, lacking adequate temporal control, may contribute to variability in diagnostic test results as well as to some of the inconsistent performance observed during aphasia therapy.

Other Forms of Temporal Alteration

Another approach to time-varying speech stimuli for use in speech
pathology and audiology entails the manual insertion of silent intervals
between the phonemic boundaries within words and between words
in phrases and sentences. Shriner and Daniloff (1970) and Beasley and
Beasley (1973) presented meaningful and non-meaningful CVC stimuli
having silent inter-phonemic intervals of 50, 100, 200, 300, and 400 ms
to first- and third-grade children. Older children performed better than
younger children and meaningful stimuli were easier than non-meaningful stimuli. Also, performance became poorer for the interphonemic
intervals greater than 100 ms, with a slight improvement in performance occurring at 400 ms. Subsequently, Beasley, Shriner, Manning and
Beasley (1974) obtained evidence that misarticulating children performed significantly poorer than normal articulating children when
presented the meaningful stimuli, but the two groups performed about
the same on the non-meaningful stimuli. Using the same materials,
Manning and Riensche (1976) obtained evidence that stuttering children performed similar to a control group of non-stuttering children,
except for superior performance of the stuttering children under the
300 ms condition. Beasley and Maki (1976) have suggested that the
pattern of changes occurring over the various interphonemic intervals
may reflect changes in processing strategies, thereby suggesting a need
for investigation of the effects of larger interphonemic intervals and a
variety of linguistic units. The stimuli appear to have diagnostic potential, but studies need to be designed to conform to normally strict
audiometric standards. For example, findings to date indicate that
sound-blending tasks which have been used to diagnose auditory processing problems in children lack sufficient temporal control to provide valid diagnostic information when administered via live-voice.

The effects of covarying word durations and interstimulus intervals
of phrases and sentences presented to adults (Aaronson, Markowitz
and Shapiro, 1971; Beasley and Shriner, 1973; Mescik *et al.*, 1972;
Kuhl and Speaks, 1972) and children (Schuckers, Shriner and Daniloff,
1973; Beasley and Flaherty-Rintelmann, 1976; Pantalos, Schuckers
and Hipskind, 1975; Schill and Schuckers, 1973; Feinberg, 1981) also
have been studied using time-sampling procedures. These investigators
have obtained evidence that the duration of both stimuli and interstimulus intervals affect performance, thereby further substantiating
the need for using controlled audiological procedures, including tape-
recorded stimuli rather than live-voice presentations, when attempting
to assess auditory processing abilities.

Summary

The preceding discussion has provided a general overview of research to date pertaining to the effects on the intelligibility and comprehension of temporally altering speech signals. Results of studies to date support the notions that reductions in the temporal redundancy of speech yield decreasing intelligibility scores in both children and adults, but that such reductions in intelligibility are age-sensitive and can be offset by increases in listening levels. Precipitous reductions in intelligibility can be expected to occur beyond about 50 per cent time compression. Research into applications of such technology to clinical populations indicates that, in addition to comparisons to normal listener scores, ear difference scores may be diagnostically relevant.

This review is not exhaustive, but rather is an attempt to encourage the reader to pursue interests in this complex area. Studies of comprehension of temporally compressed and expanded speech have been sporadic and equivocal, making it necessary for the scientific community to pursue more systematic study in this direction. Use of various modifications of linguistic structures and prosodic cues in conjunction with time alteration should provide additional important information on the temporal nature of speech perception. Equally important, such studies need to be expanded to non-native English-speaking populations (Nikam, Beasley and Rintelmann, 1976), in part because it could help clarify issues relevant to the auditory perceptual process in general, and in part because it may hold promise for universal application. The beneficial implications seem clear and the technology is available, but a great deal of detailed work lies ahead.

9 DICHOTIC LISTENING

Chris Code

Introduction

Dichotic listening was developed primarily from pioneering work by Broadbent (1954) who was among the first to discover that normal subjects tended to show a right-ear preference advantage or superiority for verbal material (Broadbent used digits) to the detriment of simultaneously presented, but different, verbal material at the left ear. The dichotic paradigm was further developed and extended to research on hemisphere asymmetries by Kimura (1961, 1967). Since this early work many dichotic studies have been carried out, and Berlin and McNeil (1976) have recently catalogued over 300 dichotic studies all using a variety of experimental procedures, stimulus materials, response methods and subjects.

The dichotic method involves the simultaneous auditory presentation of different material to the separate ears of a subject via stereophonic headphones, usually from pre-recorded tape. While one item or segment occurs at the left ear, a different item occurs at the right ear. Materials used have been typically verbal (CVC words, CV syllables, digits, etc.) or non-verbal (tonal contours, music, environmental sounds, etc.), and the general and more or less consistent finding has been that normal right-handed subjects show a right-ear preference (REP) or right-ear advantage (REA) for verbal material (Kimura, 1961, 1967; Bryden, 1963; Shankweiler and Studdert-Kennedy, 1967; Studdert-Kennedy and Shankweiler, 1970) and a left-ear preference (LEP) or left-ear advantage (LEA) for non-verbal material (Kimura, 1964; Curry, 1967; Knox and Kimura, 1970; Gordon, 1970; Haggard and Parkinson, 1971; Bryden, Ley and Sugarman, 1982; Gregory, 1982).

The overwhelmingly dominant model invoked to explain the dichotic effect is that first proposed by Kimura (1967) and illustrated in Figure 9.1. Two auditory pathways leave the inner ear: the *contralateral pathway*, which travels to the auditory area (Hescle's gyrus) in the temporal lobe of the cortical hemisphere opposite the ear, and the *ipsilateral pathway*, which runs to the auditory area in the temporal lobe of the cortical hemisphere on the same side as the ear. The contra-

Figure 9.1: The Contralateral and Ipsilateral Auditory Pathways

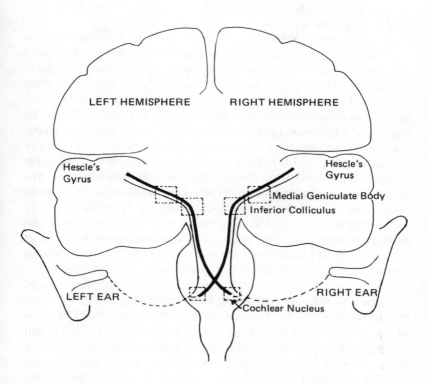

Source: Courtesy of E. Legin.

lateral pathway contains more fibres, is considered to be stronger and more efficient and is seen as inhibiting or blocking the signal travelling via the weaker ipsilateral pathway (Rosenweig, 1951; Hall and Goldstein, 1968). On this model, the observed REP for verbal material is explained as a function of the relative superiority of the left hemisphere for verbal processing and the LEP for non-verbal material as a reflection of the relative superiority of the right hemisphere for non-verbal processing.

Consequently, dichotic listening has been widely used as a comparatively simple, non-invasive technique for inferring *hemispheric* preference for various materials in a variety of populations. Studies have been carried out with subjects suffering from a variety of communication disorders, including aphasia, apraxia, dysarthria, stuttering, dyslexia, delayed and disordered language and articulation, autism and Down's syndrome, as well as others.

Among normal populations, dichotic listening has been used to examine the relationships between ear preferences (and by implication hemispheric preference) and such variables as age, sex and handedness. Bryden and Allard (1978) have concluded in their review of dichotic studies and language development that there is a 'gradual development of cerebral lateralisation which approximates the adult state by the eighth grade' (puberty) (p. 398), although there are indicators to suggest that the left hemisphere has become superior for speech perception by 5 years (Geffen, 1976; Bryden and Allard, 1978). These observations become important to questions concerned with whether left hemisphere specialisation exists at birth and does not *develop* during childhood — the 'developmental invariance' hypothesis (Kinsbourne, 1975), or whether there is bilateral hemispheric representation at birth with subsequent development of unilateral hemispheric specialisation (Lenneberg, 1967). It has also been proposed that hemispheric specialisation goes on developing and changing throughout life into old age (Brown, 1978, 1979).

The ear preferences observed in dichotic listening studies appear to be dependent upon the different phonetic characteristics of the competing stimuli (Studdert-Kennedy and Shankweiler, 1970; Darwin, 1974; Berlin and Cullen, 1977; Hayden, Kirsten and Singh, 1979; Speaks, Carney, Niccum and Johnson, 1981). Normal subjects tend to report a preference for voiceless over voiced stops, for velar place of articulation over alveolar place and for alveolar over bilabial place of articulation. Berlin and McNeil (1976) have made the point that these phonetic effects are so strong that if a dichotic tape is not properly balanced with regard to phonetic preferences, a consistent LEP could be obtained from a normal population.

Right-ear preferences have been demonstrated again and again for stop consonants but it has been more difficult to obtain significant ear preferences for vowels (Studdert-Kennedy and Shankweiler, 1970). This may be due to consonants being more 'encoded' than vowels (Liberman, Cooper, Shankweiler and Studdert-Kennedy, 1967) where consonants are seen as being perceived 'categorically' and vowels as being perceived 'continuously'. Consonant discrimination appears to be based on categorical phonetic features held in short-term memory, whereas the discrimination of vowels, which are considerably longer in duration, may be based on non-linguistic acoustic cues (Darwin, 1974). A REP for vowels has been obtained, however, by manipulating the stimuli in various ways. Weiss and House (1973) obtained a REP for vowels when white noise was added, Darwin (1971) when the vowels were produced by two different sizes (synthetic) of vocal tract and Haggard (1971) when subjects were not aware of which of two speakers would produce a particular vowel. Darwin (1971) was also able to demonstrate a REP for fricatives when they contained formant transitions. These findings have been explained by reference to acoustic memory where intelligibility is reduced by such manipulations, and decay is speeded up. A REP is obtainable because, on the acoustic memory account, it is thought that adding formant transitions causes the left-ear stimulus to fade or decay more rapidly in acoustic memory while the right-ear stimulus is being processed, thus reducing the left-ear score.

Problems exist with the size and reliability of ear differences observed in dichotic studies. Despite large *group* differences being obtained, it is often observed that the ear differences produced by *individuals* sometimes fail to reach statistical significance with the advantage to one ear over the other usually falling between 2 and 6 per cent (Schulhoff and Goodglass, 1969). Wexler, Halwes and Heninger (1981) have suggested that one-sample Chi Square analysis can be usefully employed to determine whether an individual's ear differences do in fact reach significance or what level of probability is reached.

The test-retest reliability of dichotic ear preferences is reported to be poor, with one study (Blumstein, Goodglass and Tartter, 1975) showing that nearly 30 per cent of normal subjects reversed ear preference on retest. From the clinical standpoint, it is interesting to note that brain-damaged subjects produce good test-retest reliability figures (Niccum, Rubens and Speaks, 1981), and the simpler single-report rhyming CVC word tests also report good test-retest figures (Johnson, Sommers and Weidner, 1977; Code, 1981) with normal as well as brain-damaged subjects.

Making a Dichotic Tape

Various methods are described in the literature for preparing dichotic tapes (Shankweiler and Studdert-Kennedy, 1967; Rubino, 1972; Vincent and Bradshaw, 1975; Sommers, Moore, Brady and Jackson, 1972; Code, 1981) and the interested reader is directed to Lass (1974) for a collection of many of the important studies, some of which provide detailed description of methods of construction. The method chosen will depend on the particular experimental or clinical requirements of the test as well as the level of sophistication of the equipment available.

The method to be described uses natural speech, as not only is this the simplest, but it may be the safest for determining gross preferences for 'speech'. Both natural and synthetic speech are used in dichotic tapes, with the advantage that with synthetic speech segments can be stringently controlled for duration, onset, frequency and intensity, as well as selectively manipulated for various experimental motives. Manipulations may involve staggering presentation of items, specifying degree of friction in fricatives, length in vowels and varying the transitions of formants in stops.

The procedure for constructing the tape is simplified if stereo tape recorders with moveable heads are available, but the method to be described will be the most simple requiring the minimum of specialised equipment. The method, however, is labour-intensive and requires the setting aside of plenty of uninterrupted time to produce a reliable tape of high quality.

The equipment required includes a stereophonic reel-to-reel tape recorder, two mono reel-to-reel recorders, a sound-level meter, a dual-beam storage oscilloscope, a good quality unidirectional microphone and a tape-editing kit. All tape-recorder heads must be cleaned and the two channels of the stereo machine must be checked for between-channel asymmetries before commencing. (For detailed discussion on the relative merits of different kinds of recording equipment see Chapter 1.)

It will first be necessary to decide on the type of stimulus material to be used (words, syllables, digits). For various reasons to be discussed below, a number of investigators who have completed dichotic studies with the communicatively impaired have preferred to use high frequency, CVC, simple, concrete words.

The next step is to decide on a mode of presentation. Stimuli can be presented in single pairs (one to the left and one to the right ear) with a pause between pairs to allow the subject to respond, or several pairs (typically three) can be presented in rapid succession followed by a pause for response.

Different patterns of response may be obtained depending on whether a *forced-choice* method is employed, where the subject is required to choose between one of the pairs of items presented, or *free-recall* where subjects report as many items as they can remember. *Precued partial report* is also used where the subject is required to report the item or items at the ear specified by the examiner for a given trial. Typically the subject is tapped on the left shoulder if the left-ear item is required or the right shoulder for the right-ear item. The mode of response must also be considered, especially with clinical populations who may have severe expressive difficulties. The mode can be oral, written or gestural, where the subject points to written word or digit or a picture from a multiple-choice array.

There are a number of problems with the method of presentation which requires the subject to respond to several pairs of items presented in rapid succession, especially with clinical populations where patients may have auditory retention or attention difficulties. There is evidence to suggest that an increased memory load increases the right-ear score (Yeni-Komshian and Gordon, 1974) thereby giving an artificially enhanced laterality score (Bryden and Allard, 1978). One way to eliminate possible memory effects is to require subjects to report only a single stimulus item (Studdert-Kennedy and Shankweiler, 1970). The majority of studies with aphasic subjects have used single pairs for this reason. Shanks and Ryan (1976) in their study suggest that 'an ear advantage cannot be detected on trials where both stimulus items are correctly or incorrectly perceived' (p. 102). However, other studies have shown that ear differences are enhanced when both stimulus items are reported and it is the item reported *second* which is compared across ears rather than the one reported first (Satz, Aschenbach, Pattishall and Fennell, 1965; Goodglass and Peck, 1972).

Once the stimulus material has been chosen, a complete list of pairs should be written out, ensuring that each pair occurs an equivalent number of times for each ear. For instance, if the pair 'gun — bun' is to be used six times on the tape, then the other pairs must occur six times, with one word of the pair occurring three times at each ear. The pairs must also be arranged on the tape in a quasi-random sequence and in such a way that half way through the test (after 18 presentations for a 36 item test) the head-phones can be reversed to control for any between-channel asymmetries in the playback equipment during testing.

The following method (after the test described by Starkey, 1974) uses six pairs of natural rhyming CVC words all beginning with a stop consonant. Because the method uses only six pairs of words it is relatively simple, requires less time and produces a high quality second-generation tape. The method described by Rubino (1972) is recommended (with the addition of a dual-beam storage oscilloscope) for making dichotic tapes employing CV syllables or digits. The stimulus word pairs first have to be recorded on one of the mono machines on fresh tape and the resulting tape spliced into loops, each loop bearing one pair (see Chapter 1 for advice on optimum recording conditions). Using a tape speed of 7.5 in/s it is advisable to record the pairs about 10 s apart with a gap of approximately 3 s between each member of the pair. In this way one word of the pair will be recorded, followed by a pause of 3 s, followed by the other member of the pair. This in turn is followed by about 10 s pause before the next pair. Care must be taken at this stage to record words at similar levels by reference to the VU meter of the recorder. The resulting mono tape is then spliced into separate loops, each loop containing a single word pair.

If a tape speed of 7.5 in/s has been used during recording each loop will be about 75 in long with an inter-word gap of about 22.5 in. The time gaps allowed during recording between words and between word pairs must be doubled if a tape speed of 3.75 in/s is used. Whichever is used, the resulting loops can be shortened or lengthened by splicing-in leader tape. Loops may need to be shorter or longer depending on the sizes of the mono machines used. The two mono tape recorders are then placed side by side on a bench and a chosen loop is threaded in such a way that the tape passes through the heads of both machines. The two machines are then connected to the two separate channels of the storage oscilloscope to check for simultaneity and amplitude. The recorders are switched to playback, and gradually moved closer to each other or further apart until the onsets of the two words are seen to be within ± 2 ms simultaneity on the screen of the oscilloscope. Once this has been achieved the pairs can then be recorded on a master tape. To do this, the stereo machine is loaded with a fresh tape and the outputs of the two mono machines are connected to the two separate channels of the stereo recorder.

At this stage it is again advisable to check the equivalence of the amplitudes of the two words by playing the loop through the stereo machine without recording. The amplitudes can be checked on the VU meters of the stereo machine and also by placing the dB(A) meter at the separate loudspeakers. It is advisable to use just one loudspeaker, first connected to one channel and then to the other, to avoid any possibility of asymmetries between speakers. Simply connect the speaker to channel 1 of the stereo machine, play the tape and note the displacement displayed on the dB meter. Then disconnect the speaker and connect to channel 2 to check the other word of the pair. Adjust the gain controls on the tape recorders until satisfied with the result. A maximum of 4 dB discrepancy between words is recommended.

Once satisfied with simultaneity of onset and equivalence of amplitude, two words can be recorded on fresh tape on the separate channels of the stereo machine. Once this has been done the master tape can be moved on to the next spot where it has been decided that the same pair will occur again (use a stop watch to ensure equal distance on the master tape between pairs; 10 s between pairs is usual). For a 36 item test, the pair on the loop is recorded three times on the master tape so that one word of the pair occurs at the left ear during testing. The connecting leads from the two mono machines to the stereo recorder are then switched and the pair is then recorded three times so that the *other* word of the pair occurs at the left ear during testing.

Once this simple but laborious process is complete for all pairs, a master tape of high quality is available which is only a second-generation tape. This dichotic tape can be preceded by a non-dichotic (binaural) trial tape where the individual words used in the test are presented several times in quasi-random sequence at 10 second intervals. Any number of reel-to-reel or cassette copies can be made from this master tape.

Applications in Speech Pathology and Therapeutics

Dichotic listening studies have been conducted with most groups of communication disorders as the following review shows. The approach has been most widely utilised in aphasic and stuttering populations and these studies are examined in detail.

Aphasia

A variety of response methods, stimulus materials and test lengths and difficulties have been employed in dichotic investigations with aphasic patients.

Moore and Weidner (1975) found that their control group obtained significantly higher right-ear scores (RES) than either of three aphasic subgroups classified according to months post-onset (mpo). Furthermore, the left-ear score (LES) for the controls was significantly lower than for the aphasic group. No significant difference between the mean dichotic performance was obtained for the three onset groups, although Group I (1 to 6 mpo) showed a small non-significant LEP, and Groups II (7 to 12 mpo) and III (+ 12 mpo) obtained significantly more mean correct LESs than RESs. Moore and Weidner suggest that there is a shift to the right undamaged cerebral hemisphere for language processsing which increases as a function of time post-onset.

Johnson *et al*. (1977) examined the relationship between the dichotic scores of aphasic subjects and initial severity of aphasia as determined by assessment within 4 weeks of onset of aphasia. Subjects were
also grouped into less than 6 mpo and more than 6 mpo. All twenty
controls produced the expected REP and 18 of the aphasic subjects
(N = 20) a LEP. The factor of time since onset did not reach significance,
but subjects more than 6 mpo did demonstrate a greater LEP than
subjects of less than 6 mpo. The factor of initial severity did significantly influence the results, however. The LEP scores of the initially
mild to moderate group were significantly smaller than the LEP scores
of the initially moderate to marked group. The authors interpreted
these results to mean that there was a shift to the right hemisphere for
linguistic processing which was greater in the more severely aphasic
subjects.

The factor of severity was also examined by Brady (1978) whose
results support to some extent those reported by Johnson *et al*. (1977).
He investigated the performance of five mild, five moderate and five
severe patients. The severe group showed a 37 per cent LEP, the moderate a 20 per cent LEP while the mild group produced a 28 per cent
REP, which was approximately that of the control group.

A longitudinal study has been completed (Pettit and Noll, 1979)
which measured dichotic performance and recovery in a group of subjects on two occasions separated by two months. Retest scores on
aphasia tests indicated a significant improvement although there was
much variability in individual performance. There was a significant
improvement in LESs on retest, but no significant change in RESs. This
result also was interpreted as strong support for the view that a lateral
shift takes place as the patient improves in language ability.

There have been some investigations of the dichotic responses of
different clinical types of aphasic patient. A recent study (Crosson and
Warren, 1981) compared Broca's and Wernicke's patients and found no
significant difference between the two groups. Broca's and Wernicke's
subjects both produced a significant LEP as compared to the REP of
the control group, with the Wernicke's group producing the larger, but
non-significant, LEP. Broca's subjects produced the greatest variability
in ear preferences.

Dominance and Lesion Effects

Inferring hemispheric preferences from dichotic preferences assumes
the integrity of the subject's entire auditory system, including the

primary auditory cortices of both left and right hemispheres and the interconnecting commissural pathways. A number of studies have identified and examined a *lesion effect* in the dichotic performance of brain-damaged subjects (Kimura, 1961; Sparks and Geschwind, 1968; Milner, Taylor and Sperry, 1968; Schulhoff and Goodglass, 1969; Sparks, Goodglass and Nickel, 1970; Damasio and Damasio, 1979) which should be separated from the *dominance effect*. The lesion effect tends to result in an impairment, suppression or total extinction of stimuli presented to the ear contralateral to the lesion, whereas the dominance effect produces the expected higher scores for material presented to the ear contralateral to the hemisphere specialised for processing that material (Schulhoff and Goodglass, 1969).

The earlier work observed that following the surgical removal of the left temporal lobe there was a significant suppression of right-ear scores. Additionally, some reduction in left-ear scores was seen following right temporal lobe excision. Sparks and Geschwind (1968) found a 100 per cent extinction of left-ear scores with perfect right-ear scores in a subject whose corpus callosum (the great fibre pathway linking the two hemispheres) had been surgically sectioned. This result was interpreted to mean that the callosal pathway from right temporal lobe to left temporal lobe 'is normally the most important one for reporting verbal material presented to the left ear in dichotic tasks' (Sparks and Geschwind, 1968: p. 13).

Schulhoff and Goodglass (1969) compared left-brain damaged and right-brain damaged subjects on a dichotic digit (verbal) and a dichotic musical (non-verbal) test and a 'neutral' dichotic click-counting task. On the basis of group analysis they found a bilateral decrement for material for which the damaged hemisphere is specialised. The left-brain damaged group showed a non-significant REP for digits, although six of the ten subjects actually produced a LEP. These subjects produced a near-normal performance (LEP) for music and a reduction in the RES for neutral clicks. The results for the right-brain damaged group paralleled the findings for the left-brain damaged group. There was a bilateral decrement for digits, but a clear REP. A lesion effect was not observed for music however, but click-counting showed a lesion effect with a larger deficit for the left ear.

Sparks *et al.* (1970) provide further confirmatory evidence that verbal dichotic information travels from left ear to right temporal lobe and thence to left temporal lobe via the corpus callosum and from right ear to left temporal lobe via the auditory pathways. On this interpretation, a left-hemisphere lesion can impede stimuli from the left ear via the corpus callosum, whereas a right hemisphere lesion can only affect a stimulus which has arrived directly from the left ear to the right temporal lobe via the auditory pathway. A diagrammatical representation of this model is shown in Figure 9.2.

Figure 9.2: The Model Proposed by Sparks *et al.* (1970) to Explain Extinction of Dichotic Stimuli in Brain-damaged Patients. The broken lines represent the ipsilateral pathways and the areas L1, L2, L3, R1 and R2 represent the sites of lesions which can produce extinction.

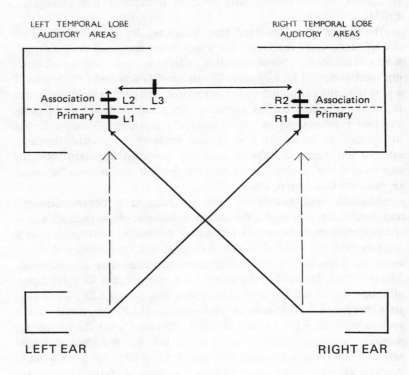

Source: Reprinted with permission from Sparks *et al.* (1970).

Damasio and Damasio (1979) have extended the dichotic paradigm to map in some detail the probable interhemispheric auditory pathway

via the corpus callosum. They did this by comparing dichotic performance with actual lesion sites detected by computerised axial tomography (CAT) scans. To summarise their findings briefly, left ear
extinction was found to be associated with lesions in the left and
right posterior parieto-occipital and right mid-temporal region; and
right ear extinction was related to lesions in the left temporal and
right parieto-occipital regions. Subjects who obtained 'normal' ear
preferences had lesions in the right frontal, left frontal and left posterior occipital region. The authors conclude that left-ear extinction
in brain-damaged subjects is associated with a lesion at any point
along the course of the interhemispheric auditory pathway, irrespec-
tive of hemisphere. This must run, they argue, from the geniculo-
cortical pathways posteriorly and upwards to arch around the lateral
ventricles joining the posterior region of the corpus callosum.

The studies which have identified and examined the lesion effect
in brain-damaged patients raise the important question as to how
much credibility can be given to dichotic investigations with aphasic
patients which have interpreted ear preference scores as indicative
of a shift in hemispheric preference, as a function of time since-onset,
severity, or type of aphasia.

The indications are that the ear preferences produced by aphasic
patients are determined by a combination of site of lesion (lesion
effect) *and* hemispheric preference (dominance). However, it may
be possible to separate these effects in dichotic listening. The fore-
going review suggests that the most consistent and robust result obtained is the increase in LEP scores over REP scores as a function
of time since-onset. Studies which have examined other variables such
as severity and type of aphasia have produced inconsistent results
which can unfortunately be explained just as well in terms of lesion
effects. The lesion effect cannot explain the increase in LEP scores
as a function of time since-onset however, nor does it explain why
patients with anterior lesions (non-fluent aphasia), presumably with
intact auditory cortex, should show a LEP. This is not to ignore the
probable intimate relationship between the anterior (Broca's) and
posterior (Wernicke's) areas. As Crosson and Warren (1981) have
also pointed out, a lesion in the anterior area might interfere with
the processing capabilities of the posterior area such that dichotic
performance could be affected. Even so, current knowledge might
indicate that non-fluent patients showing a LEP are demonstrating
a genuine shift in hemispheric preference for verbal material, especially if this LEP can be shown to increase with time since-onset.

A recent study (Code, 1983a) attempted to examine this question. The ear preferences of 27 aphasic subjects grouped into fluent (posterior) and non-fluent (anterior) were compared on a simple CVC word test. Results revealed highly significant increases in LESs and decreases in RESs in non-fluent subjects who were more than 12 months post-onset than non-fluent subjects who were less than 12 months post-onset. Significant differences were not found, however, in fluent subjects who were less than and more than 12 months post-onset. Such results may suggest that for non-fluent subjects with anterior damage and intact posterior mechanisms, superior LESs may reflect an increased involvement of the right hemisphere in verbal processing (dominance effect), but for fluent subjects with damage to posterior auditory processing mechanisms, dichotic responses reflect a lesion effect and cannot be reliably interpreted in terms of hemispheric shift. It could be that a lesion effect may mask any dominance effect in posteriorly damaged patients. However, this interpretation assumes that posterior mechanisms are unaffected by anterior damage, and this may be too simplistic and unrealistic a characterisation of the relationship between anterior and posterior mechanisms.

The results are in general agreement with those reported recently by Castro-Caldas and Botelho (1980) who tested 117 aphasic subjects on three dichotic tests. In both a retrospective and longitudinal analysis, non-fluent patients showed a tendency towards a left-ear preference with time since-onset and fluent subjects a tendency towards right-ear preference with time since-onset.

Further longitudinal studies are required to examine the relationship between changes in ear preference and recovery in different aphasic groups.

Stuttering

Dichotic listening has been used to examine the hypothesis first advanced by Orton (1928) and Travis (1931) that cerebral organisation in stutterers is in some way different from that of non-stutterers. Some of the major studies will be discussed.

Curry and Gregory (1969) compared 20 adult stutterers and 20 adult non-stutterers on a dichotic CVC word test, a dichotic environmental sound test and a dichotic pitch test. Both groups showed the expected REP for the word test, although the REP was statistically significant only for the non-stutterers. No differences were obtained between the two groups on either the environmental sound or pitch tests. However, when the size of the absolute between-ears difference scores were compared, a highly significant superiority was observed for the control group. Moreover, 11 (55 per cent) of the stutterers actually showed a LEP on the word test which was masked by the group analysis. It was also reported that a number of those stutterers (73 per cent) producing a LEP showed a REP for one or other of the non-verbal tests. These results may be interpreted as support for the hypothesis that stutterers have incomplete or bilateral hemispheric representation for verbal processing.

Brady and Berson (1975) conducted an examination of the dichotic performance of 35 adult stutterers and a matched group of controls, all carefully assessed to be right-handed. The stutterers were classified as severe. The CVC test developed by Shankweiler and Studdert-Kennedy (1967) was used in this study where subjects responded by circling one of the two written nonsense syllables. Results showed that all controls produced the expected REP with six (17 per cent) of the stutterers producing a LEP which failed to reach significance. No differences in severity or sex were apparent between the LEP and REP subgroups of stutterers. Stutterers also showed smaller between-ear differences than non-stutterers. The study concludes that there may be a subset of stutterers whose brain organisation is different.

Dorman and Porter (1975) used a slightly different test to Brady and Berson (1975) in their group comparison of 16 right-handed moderate/severe adult stutterers and 20 controls. The test used 120 single-pair presentations of synthetic CV syllables and subjects responded by writing both syllables down. Male stutterers and male and female non-stutterers produced a significant REP on the test, but female stutterers as a group (N = 4) did not, although three of these subjects did produce large REP scores. No significant differences between stutterers and non-stutterers emerged in this group analysis and the authors suggest that there is no support for the Orton-Travis theory.

Rosenfield and Goodglass (1980) conducted a study which attempted to avoid some of the methodological shortcomings of earlier studies in the hope of producing more unequivocal results. They restricted the study to well-matched male stutterers and controls and examined non-verbal ear preferences with Kimura's (1964) dichotic melodies test. The verbal test was a natural CV syllable single-pair test which required written report of both syllables. Order of report was also controlled for by the examiner tapping subjects on either right or left shoulder before each pair. Each subject was required to write down first the CV syllable corresponding to the side which had been tapped.

As has been mentioned in an earlier section, studies have shown that ear differences are enhanced when the stimulus which is reported *second* is compared across ears rather than the first (Satz *et al.*, 1965; Goodglass and Peck, 1972). The investigators also conducted a retest for all subjects one week after the first testing to compare stability of preferences in the groups. Group analysis of the degree of REP showed no differences between the two groups on the CV test. Controls produced a greater difference between ears on the stimuli reported second than on those reported first, in agreement with previous studies. However, the stuttering groups produced the opposite result — ear differences on the stimuli reported first were greater than those reported second. This pattern for stutterers and non-stutterers was repeated on retest. On examining the consistency of *individual* subjects between test and retests it was found that subjects in both groups changed ear preference on retest on the verbal task, but the proportion of control subjects who showed consistent REP was greater than stutterers. Over 25 per cent of stutterers produced a consistent LEP. Group analysis showed that non-stutterers and stutterers showed a LEP for the musical test. Individual results on test and retest revealed that consistency between the two tests for both groups was poor, but worse for the stutterers.

These results suggest 'abnormal' lateralisation for verbal and non-verbal material for a subgroup of stutterers which would support the Orton-Travis theory, as although group analysis revealed no differences, the individual performances of some stutterers showed marked deviations.

Allen (1980) using a synthetic CV syllable test, has recently produced evidence to support the notion that there are two distinct subgroups of stutterers and that an individual stutterer's ear-preference score is related to the severity of the disorder. Three groups, each made up of 24 right-handed subjects were tested. The groups were severe stutterers, moderate/mild stutterers and non-stutterers. Severity was determined by a combination of percentage of words stuttered per minute and number of words spoken per minute. Results showed that severe stutterers do produce significantly different ear preferences to milder stutterers and normal subjects.

It was indicated earlier that the dichotic listening paradigm constitutes a *perceptual* task. Consequently direct inferences about hemispheric processing of speech *production* or expression cannot legitimately be made. In conventional dichotic studies, the most that can be claimed is that ear preferences may reflect a hemispheric perceptual preference, even in those studies using oral report. Sussman and Mac-Neilage (1975) developed a method which they considered measured hemispheric perceptual and production processes. They combined a dichotic listening task with a paradigm they called *pursuit auditory tracking* to compare language lateralisation in adult stutterers and non-stutterers. The procedure required the subject to match a tone in one ear with a tone in the second ear. The tone in the second ear varied randomly in frequency and amplitude under computer control. The subject could manipulate the tone in the first ear by movement of the jaw or tongue. This movement was transformed into signals which variated the tone in the first ear so that the subject could attempt to match up the tones. Sussman and MacNeilage argue that pursuit auditory tracking is capable of measuring hemispheric involvement in speech production. A comparison of stutterers and non-stutterers on this combined paradigm showed that non-stutterers as a group were more adept at the articulatory task (i.e. non-stutterers were better at manipulating the right ear tone to match the randomly variated tone in the left ear). This was interpreted as a REP (left-hemisphere preference) for speech production in non-stutterers. Stutterers did not show such a preference which suggests that, as a group, the stutterers demonstrated less left-hemisphere superiority for perception and production than the normal group. However, a subgroup again emerged whose hemispheric superiority matched that of the non-stutterers confirming a consistently observed finding that some stutterers do perform as if they were less lateralised for language processing.

Some studies have examined dichotic preferences in stuttering children. Gruber and Powell (1974) found no significant differences between 28 stuttering and 28 non-stuttering children using a test employing the presentation of digits in sets of three. The ages of the children ranged from 8 years 5 months to 18 years 8 months. Furthermore, neither group produced significant inter-ear differences, confirming those studies (Kimura, 1963) that have found no differences in normal children.

In contrast, Sommers, Brady and Moore (1975) in their comparison of right-handed stuttering and non-stuttering children and adults obtained different results. This study examined dichotic word and digit performance of 78 subjects, between the ages of 4½ and 48 years and classified into three age groups, with 13 stutterers in each group. The dichotic word test consisted of four pairs of CVC rhyming words and the digit test of four pairs of digits. A single-pair presentation oral-report method was used with all subjects. Results on the word test showed that non-stutterers produced larger ear-preference scores, a larger proportion of stutterers failed to show a REP and only 16 of the 39 stutterers across all three age groups produced a REP. On the digit test nine non-stutterers and 17 stutterers failed to produce a REP and nine stutterers across all age groups produced a LEP score. Excluding the effect of age, no differences were found for non-stutterers, but stuttering children produced significantly lower REP scores than stuttering adults.

These results again support the finding that separate subgroups of stutterers exist, some of whom may have a lack of lateralisation for linguistic processing or bilateral representation. The authors also speculate that the spontaneous remission of stuttering in older children may have something to do with the development of speech perception or the establishment of hemispheric dominance, and that these functions may be slower to develop in stutterers.

Some consistent trends appear to emerge from an inspection of the research on dichotic listening in stutterers. Studies which have examined individual scores more closely have found that there are grounds for believing in the existence of two distinct subgroups: one which shows ear preferences similar to non-stutterers and one which does not. There are some indications that severity of stuttering and age may be related to this finding. It would appear that the variables of sex and handedness (particularly familiar left-handedness) need to be examined in future studies. These variables have not been examined closely in studies to date and may contribute to the inconsistency in findings.

Other Disorders

Dichotic studies have been completed with a range of other speech, language and learning disordered groups relevant to speech pathology, including dyslexic and poor reading children and adults, language disordered and articulation disordered children, and minimal brain-damaged and Down's syndrome children. Some of these studies will be briefly discussed.

Dichotic investigations of individuals with reading disability have been comprehensively reviewed by Satz (1976) showing that results have been equivocal with some studies demonstrating a REP in such groups and other studies failing to produce significant ear preferences. The issues are discussed by Beaumont and Rugg (1978) and Wilsher (1981). Witelson (1976, 1977) used dichotic digits and visual tactile tests to examine lateral preference in dyslexic children. Her results indicated that such children demonstrate left-hemisphere preference for verbal material, but right-hemisphere preference for non-verbal material. This led her to suggest that dyslexia is due to a disfunction of the right hemisphere, imposing extra non-verbal responsibilities on the left. The left becomes overloaded, responsible as it is for verbal and non-verbal processing, and its verbal efficiency is reduced. Support for Witelson's hypothesis has been supplied recently by Newell and Rugel (1981). Using dichotic melodies and digits they found a REP for digits in normal and disabled readers, but disabled readers also produced a REP for music in contrast to the LEP found in the normal group.

The opposing view, that dyslexia represents a right-hemisphere specialisation for language has received some support from dichotic studies by Chasty (1979, 1981). Using four sets of digits he obtained a LEP in dyslexic children, which he suggests reflects a less efficient neurological organisation for language for such children. (As in other areas of dichotic research, comparisons between studies are precarious due to such factors as design differences, dichotic test differences and subject criteria.) In contrast, a three-pair dichotic digit study of illiterate adults (Tzavaras, Kaprinis and Gatzoyas, 1981) showed a highly superior REP with near extinction of the left ear, suggesting that reading and writing skills in *educated* adults involve considerable right-hemisphere involvement.

A series of studies conducted by Sommers and associates have examined ear preferences in a range of speech and language disordered children. Most of these studies have used the simple single CVC rhyming word pair test described in the introduction to this chapter. The Sommers and Taylor (1972) study which examined the ear preferences of speech and language delayed children used a two and three-pair digit test. These children produced significantly greater LEP scores in contrast to the control group's significantly better REP. Sommers *et al.* (1972) compared the performance of normal, mild articulation disordered, severely articulation disordered and minimally brain-damaged articulation disordered children on the single-pair word test. They found a relationship between severity and ear preference. The more severe the articulation problem, the greater the tendency towards a LEP for words; the severe group produced no ear preferences suggesting a lack of left-hemisphere specialisation for language.

Sommers and Starkey (1977) investigated the ear preferences of Down's syndrome children in a high speech and language performance and a low speech and language performance group. Controls produced the expected REP but both groups of Down's syndrome subjects failed to produce any ear preference. Examinations of the phonetic effects of the test showed that the high performance group tended to produce similar phonetic preferences to the normal group, but the low performance group tended to produce different phonetic preferences. This is in contrast to the result produced by Hartley (1981) recently, who found a LEP in 11 young Down's syndrome female subjects. Hartley used a single-syllable 38 word-pair test with oral report.

Prior and Bradshaw (1979) examined the performance of 19 autistic children on a 24 single-syllable word-pair test. They found considerable variability in results, with five subjects showing a REP, seven a LEP and the remaining seven no ear preference. There were correlations also between ear preferences and the presence or absence of speech before the age of 5 years as well as a relation with IQ level. The authors suggest that the LEP group may have developed right-hemisphere dominance for language.

Clinical Applications

Dichotic listening is an experimental paradigm about which there is considerable uncertainty. Information is slowly emerging concerning stimulus material, test length, response method and the power of dichotic listening to tap and measure hemispheric preference for auditory perception. Already there are clinics which use dichotic listening as a simple non-invasive method for investigating hemispheric preference on a routine basis, although it is clear that there are a number of questions concerning general reliability which remain to be answered. Bearing this in mind, the state of the art is such that dichotic listening is a useful non-invasive, relatively simple and cheap technique, the results of which especially with the brain-damaged need to be supplemented by other forms of investigation. With current knowledge it is safer to suggest that the technique can only have a contributory role.

We have seen that there are indications that dichotic listening may have a contributory role in the future as a non-invasive method for localising lesions. In the management of aphasia, the planning of treatment methods which are designed to utilise the undamaged hemisphere (Buffery and Burton, 1982; Code, 1983b) can be aided by dichotic assessment. More information can be obtained if non-verbal as well as verbal dichotic processing is assessed and tachistoscopic hemifield viewing might be utilised to supplement dichotic results (Linebaugh, 1978). At the present time however, dichotic listening is predominantly an experimental technique, and its general clinical application remains to be determined more fully.

Therapeutic Applications

There are, as yet, few reports of the application of dichotic listening in the actual treatment of communication disorders. However, it would appear that there is much scope for the development of such treatment methods. The experiment described by Code (1983b) employed specially made dichotic tapes to direct material to the undamaged right hemisphere of a Wernicke's aphasic patient in an attempt specifically to improve auditory comprehension. One to three pairs of digits were employed to increase auditory memory span and dichotically contrasting CV syllables were used to improve phonemic discrimination. Dichotic and tachistoscopic methods were also combined in a cross-model programme. The results of the experiment were mixed in so far as the patient improved dramatically on digit retention and other specific areas, but made only modest improvement in general communicative ability as determined by aphasia battery assessment. The results were considered promising however, and indicated that the method should be examined further.

A number of possible innovations would appear to be worthy of investigation. Where assessment has indicated that an aphasic patient may be using the right hemisphere, comprehension material might be presented in dichotic competition with instructions to attend to the left ear. Performance could then be compared to instructions to attend to the right ear, and binaural presentation. This could conceivably be done with digits, syllables and words as well as sentences and longer comprehension passages. Material might be presented within the same experimental framework in a musical context to see whether combining verbal stimuli with material, known to be processed more efficiently by the right hemisphere ('priming' the right hemisphere) improves performance.

From the review of studies in this Chapter it is clear that relationships have been inferred between neuropsychological dysfunction or abnormality and a range of communication disorders. It would seem logical therefore, for those concerned with the treatment of such disorders, to consider the possibilities of employing techniques like dichotic listening, possibly in combination with tachistoscopic viewing. For specific disorders which may be characterised by difficulties in deriving sound from print, for instance, a combined dichotic-tachistoscopic method could be designed which could direct material to just one or to both hemispheres (dichotic to one, tachistoscopic to the other).

Conclusion

We have examined in some detail the major dichotic studies that have been carried out with individuals exhibiting a variety of communication disorders. We have spent more time considering those studies in aphasia and stuttering as other areas are less well developed. A number of conclusions emerge. Firstly, it is clear that many investigators feel that ear preferences which differ from those of normal control groups reflect a different neurocognitive organisation in many groups. The above review indicates that different neurocognitive organisation, whether right-hemisphere dominance, bilateral representation, disordered or inefficient interhemispheric transmission, has been proposed as a major contributory factor in many human communication disorders. Indeed, the disorder which does not have such neurocognitive abnormalities as part of its underlying aetiology, would appear on the basis of the interpretations made of dichotic results, to be a very rare phenomenon!

We have seen also that it is by no means certain that there is a cause and effect relationship between ear-preference scores and hemispheric preference, that the reliability of dichotic tests is such that some 30 per cent of subjects may reverse their preferences on retest (with some tests) and that brain damage will cause ear preferences which may have more to do with the nature and site of the lesion than with the hemispheric preference for particular kinds of material.

The above review has also shown that a number of response modes have been used in dichotic studies as well as a variety of materials. Furthermore, subject selection criteria have been different, as well as analysis of results. While researchers will continue to adopt the methods which appear most appropriate to them, the lack of consistency between studies with regard to these critical variables makes comparison of results difficult and replication with 'non-normal' groups disappointing.

Clearly a great deal more research is required to establish the most appropriate forms of dichotic tests and the best methods of administration for clinical use which are reliable and valid measures of hemispheric preference for various aspects of language.

10 ORAL STEREOGNOSIS

Steven E. Deutsch

Introduction

The production of oral communication requires highly complex planning and coordination of movement which is responsible for the generation and valving of the breath stream for speech. Together the muscles and structures which valve the breath stream comprise the motor subsystems of respiration, phonation, resonance and articulation. The complexity of the motor coordination required for speech is illustrated by Lenneberg's (1967) estimation that more than 100 muscles must be sequentially or concurrently innervated in order to activate the motor subsystems noted above. Furthermore, Darley *et al*. (1975) calculated that a single second of speech produced at an average rate of 14 phonemes per second requires approximately 140,000 neuromuscular events. In the presence of such complexity various theories and models have been proposed in attempts to help explain numerous aspects of speech behaviour.

A number of theories are based on servosystem models. In general, servosystem models incorporate feedback that may be used to monitor, regulate and modify the output of the overall system. In terms of speech, both auditory and somaesthetic components of feedback have been proposed. Fairbank's (1954) model of oral motor control incorporated sensory monitoring of motor activity. The result of this monitored activity was incorporated in a comparison of the output with the input for the purpose of detecting and measuring errors. Subsequently, appropriate adjustments could be made, resulting in a match of the output to the input. Liberman's (1957) 'motor theory' of speech perception is predicated upon the supposition that an acoustic stimulus leads to a covert articulatory response. Although this articulatory response is highly similar to that used during production, during perception, the listener associates speech sounds with their corresponding articulatory movements. Neural activity associated with these covert articulatory movements is fed back and serves as a mediator between the acoustic stimulus and its eventual perception. Henke's (1967) perspective on speech production stressed the importance of sensory feedback. He proposed that proprioceptive feedback provides the mechanism for the control of timing or rate of articulatory movements. A variety of different types of feedback including acoustic, myotactic, air pressure and tactile were incorporated into Perkell's (1969) perspective of the speech production mechanism. MacNeilage (1970) in his discussion of the serial ordering of speech referred to the role of somaesthetic, kinaesthetic and auditory feedback. He suggested that during language development these forms of feedback may assist in the acquisition of internal spatial representation of target positions within the oral cavity. Although a single definitive model of speech production has yet to be identified, a sensory feedback component is present in the majority of models proposed thus far (Mlcoch and Noll, 1980).

The clinical literature has also acknowledged the possible role of sensory feedback during speech production. Specifically, suggestions have been made regarding the need to assess tactile and kinaesthetic sensitivity in the oral region during diagnosis (Emerick and Hatten, 1974). Similarly, treatment approaches have alluded to the possible importance of oral sensory perception. Van Riper and Irwin (1958) suggested a remediation approach based upon the eventual dependence of kinaesthetic and/or tactile cues for speech monitoring. McDonald (1964) emphasised the use of oral sensory processes by recommending that a patient describe the speech movements and articulatory contacts produced in various combinations of sound contexts. Additionally, efforts to improve palatal function have employed training techniques designed to increase kinaesthetic awareness of velar positioning (Van Riper, 1954; Berry and Eisenson, 1957; Shelton, Knox, Elbert and Johnson, 1970; Shprintzen, McCall and Skolnick, 1975).

In addition to clinical suggestions, a number of research studies have been focused on the ability of both normal and speech-defective subjects to detect and utilise information obtained through the oral sensory receptive mode. Tasks studied have included: two-point discrimination (Ringel and Ewanowski, 1965; McCall and Morgan, 1967; McCall and Cunningham, 1971; Lass, Kotchek and Deem, 1972; Lass and Park, 1973); oral texture discrimination (Ringel and Fletcher, 1967); tactile extinction (McCall, 1965, 1966); mandibular kinaesthesis (Ringel, Saxman and Brooks, 1967); palatal kinaesthesis (Shelton, Beaumont, Trier and Furr, 1978; Shelton *et al.*, 1970); threshold for vibrotactile stimuli (Fucci, Hall and Weiner, 1971; Telage and Fucci, 1973, 1974); tactile acuity, localisation, discrimination pattern recognition and kinaesthetic pattern recognition (Rutherford and McCall,

1967). The findings of these studies suggest that oral sensory function and the information it provides is relevant to speech production and possibly remediation. However, the scope of the present chapter will be limited to that body of literature concerned with the specific aspect of oral sensory function associated with oral stereognosis.

Definition of Oral Stereognosis

Stereognosis is literally defined as the ability to recognise the shape or form of objects by manual palpation or manipulation without the benefit of vision (Chusid, 1973). Forster (1962) suggests that tests of stereognosis should be included in a neurological examination as an indicator of nervous system integrity. Paine (1967) pointed out that the general clinical administration of such tests requires the patient to identify such common objects as a key, coin or paper clip. Correct performance on this task requires more than the simple detection of tactile attributes. In addition, it requires higher cortical activities likely involving the integration and association of afferent sensations with the criterial attributes of the test object. Clearly, an impairment either at the level of peripheral reception or cortical integration may be responsible for an impairment in stereognosis. The term astereognosis implies a total inability to perform stereognostic tasks. However, it also is used as a reference to a partial deficit, rather than a complete inability.

An expansion of the clinical application of stereognosis testing to include oral structures was proposed by Critchley (1953). He described the possibility of testing oral sensation utilising an oral stereognosis task. For the purposes of the present discussion, oral stereognosis will refer to the ability to identify objects through oral exploration employing any of the procedural variations to be discussed later. An additional term 'oral form recognition' will be used synonomously with oral stereognosis. The former term is favoured by the present author when the procedure employs specially designed sets of geometric forms which do not require prior experience with the object.

Possible Neurological Bases of Oral Stereognosis

Correct performance on an oral stereognosis task requires successful completion of two sensorineural processes. First, the sensory perceptual system extracts the sensory detail from the stimulus object which is resting or being manipulated in the oral cavity. Second, cognitive processing of the sensory information takes place which results in either a discriminative identification or, matching of the stimulus to a model form. At present we do not have detailed understanding of the mechanisms responsible for the detection and transmission of the sensory information, and we have even more speculative notions regarding the cognitive processing of this information. Nevertheless, it has been suggested that stereognosis is dependent on integration of the sensations of touch-pressure and kinaesthesis (Mountcastle and Darian-Smith, 1968; Grossman, 1967).

Tactile Sensations

During an oral stereognostic task, the stimulus form is placed on the tongue. Such placement likely results in tactile sensations even prior to active oral exploration of the object by the subject being tested. First, it is likely that the sensation of simple touch occurs. This sensation includes light touch and pressure as well as a crude sense of localisation (Clark, 1975). Second, a more specific tactile component is usually noted and variously labelled by different authors. These more specific sensations include the sense of pressure gradient and specific spatial location of pressure. Such sensations may be useful in two-point discrimination and detection of size and shape of the stimulus object. Both types of tactile sensation may arise from structures other than the tongue since during oral stereognostic tasks the stimulus form is manipulated and explored inside the mouth. Grossman and Hattis (1967) identified numerous forms of neural receptors which are responsible for various tactile sensations arising from the oral mucosa. These included capsulated and non-capsulated organised endings, fibrillar extensions, nerve networks, free nerve endings and simple and complex branched terminations. Information from these receptors is transmitted via the trigeminal lemniscal system to the thalamus and eventually bilaterally projected to somaesthetic areas of the cortex. Thus, when an oral stereognosis form is placed in a subject's mouth, these various tactile receptors contribute a variety of information used for identification or matching. However, depending upon the size, shape complexity and weight of the stimulus object, more than just tactile sensations may be required to perform the stereognostic task. Additional sensory input from kinaesthetic receptors derived during oral exploration may be necessary.

Kinaesthesis

Kinaesthesis refers to those somaesthetic sensations which result in an awareness of body position and movement (Smith, Roberts and Atkins, 1972; Frank, Williams and Hayes, 1977; Kelso, 1977). Information derived from kinaesthesis may be utilised in the oral stereognosis task in at least two ways. First, it provides a form of feedback involved in movement control of the oral structures during oral exploration and manipulation of the stimulus form. Such oral manipulation involves tongue and lip movements and variations in jaw opening. Second, kinaesthetic sensations probably assist in the extraction of somaesthetic information which occurs when a subject traces the outline of a form with the tongue. During these exploratory tracing movements, some persisting sensory image may be extracted which describes the movement of the oral structures around the perimeter of the object. This image may eventually allow recognition of the object through its outline representation. In addition, Hardy (1970) defined kinaesthesia to include sensory feedback of the relative position of structures and rates of changes in positions. This information may also help in discerning the size of the object.

This complex array of kinaesthetic sensation is detected by such structures as joint receptors, Golgi tendon organs, and muscle spindles. The importance of these proprioceptors to speech production has been demonstrated by studies which disrupted sensory feedback and produced impaired articulation and intelligibility (McCroskey, 1958; McCroskey, Corley and Jackson, 1959; Ringel and Steer, 1963; Schliesser and Coleman, 1968). However, relatively little specific information is available concerning the role of kinaesthetic receptors in oral stereognosis. Nevertheless, both Gibson's (1962) data on active versus passive touch and Shelton, Arndt and Hetherington's (1967) comprehensive discussion suggest that kinaesthesis is probably of particular importance in stereognostic perception. The present discussion will focus on those receptors most likely to participate in oral kinaesthesis.

Receptors Involved in Kinaesthesis. Joint receptors are specialised structures probably involved in the perception of joint position. They are embedded within the sheath surrounding a joint and are located in that portion of the joint which is stretched maximally during movement. They include such structures as Ruffini endings and Pacinian corpuscles. Reports by Boyd and Roberts (1953), Burgess and Clark (1969) and Smith (1977) indicate the complexity of the role of joint receptors in the perception of joint position. Specifically, it has been determined that the firing pattern of joint receptors is dependent on such factors as extremes of joint movement, active versus passive movement, and the direction of motion. The Golgi tendon organ is a second type of receptor for the perception of movement information. It has been shown to respond to stretch placed on a muscle with an inhibitory reaction resulting in a decrease of muscle tension. These stretch receptors are located between the contractile elements in the muscle and the tendon that attaches the muscle to the bone. Therefore, they appear to be ideally located to provide information about tension in the muscles via their connections by I_b sensory fibres to the central nervous system. Evidence presented by Houk and Henneman (1967) and Stuart, Mosher, Gerlack and Reinking (1972) indicated that the attachment ratio of tendon organs to muscle fibres and motor units is quite small. This innervation ratio permits detection of muscular tension which may exist in specific localised portions of a particular muscle as innervated by different motor units.

The muscle spindle is a third type of specialised proprioceptor. It is composed of from two to ten specialised muscle fibres (intrafusal fibres) which are encapsulated in a fusiform structure and attached at both ends and in parallel to the regular muscle fibres (extrafusal fibres). As a result of its attachment to the main muscle, the spindle is subjected to stretch whenever the muscle is stretched. This stretch information detected by the spindle is transmitted via the muscle spindle afferent to the spinal cord where it synapses directly with the alpha motor neurone resulting in contraction of the same muscle. This mechanism provides the basis for the simple stretch reflex which results in quick unsustained phasic movement.

Additionally, the muscle spindle has a prominent role in the maintenance of sustained, postural, tonic aspects of movement, which are more likely involved in the sensory feedback and movement control requirements of an oral form recognition task. The gamma motor system, utilising multisynaptic chains of neurones, is responsible for this function. The intrafusal fibres of the spindle are innervated by small gamma motor neurones which may receive their stimulation via peripheral tactile afferents or from subcortical and cortical structures. The resultant change in spindle length can be perceived by I_a afferent fibres that are attached to the central region of the spindle and transmit information about the length and rate of change of muscle length to the spinal cord segment or to higher sensory regions of the cortex (Goodwin, McCloskey and Matthews, 1972a, b).

At the spinal cord the sensory impulses synapse with the alpha motor neurone which then discharges directly to the main muscle fibres causing them to contract until they match the length of the muscle

spindle. These inputs to and from the muscle spindle serve to prepare
for the muscle contraction requirements of a particular movement and
therefore play a considerable role in the movement regulation required
during oral exploration of a stereognosis form (see Figure 10.1).

**Figure 10.1: Muscle Spindle Responsible for Stretch Reflex and Activity
of the Gamma Loop**

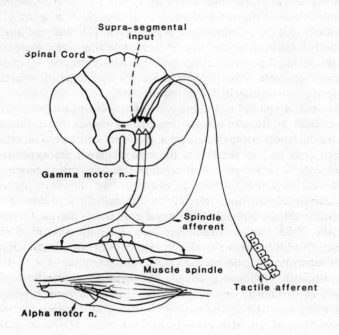

All of the above receptors are involved in kinaesthesis. Proprioceptive fibre collaterals primarily from I_a and I_b afferents enter at the level
of the brain stem and may diverge in at least three routes. They may
become part of the gamma-alpha loop involved in reflex activity.
Alternatively, these fibres may contribute proprioceptive information
for movement control at an unconscious level via cerebellar pathways.
Specifically, several authors reported that information from muscle
spindles is relayed to the cerebellum and not the sensory cortex (Rose
and Mountcastle, 1959; Rutherford and McCall, 1967; Boyd, Eyzaguirre, Matthews and Rushworth, 1968). Thirdly, recent evidence

(Goodwin, McCloskey and Matthews, 1972a) suggests that at least a portion of the I_a and I_b fibres may become part of the lemniscal system and eventually pass to the post central gyrus somaesthetic areas of the cortex.

Additional processing of the cerebellar and cortical level information was discussed by Wetzel and Stuart (1976). They suggest the ensemble of sensory information from joint receptors, tendon organs and muscle spindles is disambiguated by the central nervous system to result in a kinaesthetic awareness.

Unfortunately, the majority of the neurophysiological research regarding kinaesthesis has not employed bulbar musculature and structures. The above statement notwithstanding, the function of kinaesthetic feedback in oral structure movement control and sensory perception depends on the documented presence of the appropriate receptors and their suitable connections to the central nervous system. Specifically, the tongue, lips and palate have been considered to have a questionable role in kinaesthesis in view of conflicting research findings concerning the presence of these sensory receptors. Of these three structures, the tongue is of particular relevance with regard to oral stereognosis tasks, since it is typically used to explore the outline and surface of the stimulus form. Although debate exists concerning the presence or absence of muscle spindles in the tongue (Cooper, 1953; Blom, 1960; Kawamura, 1970), further evidence (Bowman, 1971) suggests that the tongue does contain muscle spindles. Furthermore, these spindles are differentially sensitive to stretch imposed from transverse, vertical, and horizontal directions. Thus, the following expansion of Sussman's (1972) conclusion appears reasonable; that the combined information transmitted from muscle spindles and tactile receptors in the tongue, as well as joint receptors in the mandible, all contribute to the coordinated control of oral structure movements and position sense involved in oral stereognosis.

Oral Stereognosis in Speech Pathology

Despite the lack of definitive information regarding neurophysiological mechanisms that underlie oral somaesthesis, considerable energy has been devoted toward the development and refinement of formal procedures for the assessment of oral stereognosis. These efforts have focused upon documenting differences in oral form recognition performance as a function of procedural variations, subject age and type of communication disorder present.

Procedural Variations

Much of the early research directed toward the development of formal tests of oral stereognosis was initiated by Eugene McDonald (McDonald and Aungst, 1967). McDonald's interest in this area was a logical extension of his sensory motor approach to articulation testing and treatment (McDonald, 1964). His research and that of others was reported at two symposia on oral sensation and perception (Bosma, 1967, 1970). These volumes include studies which reported the effects of various test paradigms, stimulus forms and efforts to develop a standardised test of oral stereognosis. It was the underlying intent of these efforts to document a correlation between oral stereognosis and both developing speech proficiency among normals and degree of articulatory deficit in speech-defective subjects.

Smith (1964) employed 15 oral stereognostic forms to test 25 speech-defective children. The forms included ten provided by the National Institute of Dental Research (NIDR) plus five three-dimensional items (Figures 10.2a rows one and two and 10.2b). As a preliminary qualification procedure, subjects were required visually to match a form held up by the examiner to an identical item positioned within an array of all 15 forms. After it was determined that the child could perform this visual matching test, one form attached to a length of dental floss was placed inside the child's mouth without the benefit of visual inspection. The child was able to manipulate the object without a time limit until he could point to its identical match from the visual array. All forms were presented singly and in random order. Results of this procedure indicated that the task contained predominantly easy items correctly identified by most of the children. This resulted in a poorly discriminating measure of oral stereognostic ability for these subjects in this test paradigm.

A more difficult and expanded set of forms was used by Aungst (1965) to test 80 kindergarten and first grade children. These forms include those previously used by Smith (1964) and ten additional forms developed by the NIDR (Figure 10.2a rows three and four). Aungst (1965) employed the same matching paradigm used by Smith (1964). The results indicated that some items were indeed more difficult than others and approximately 97 per cent of the variance in total test scores could be accounted for by a general factor identified as oral stereognosis. Aungst compared his subjects' preliminary visual matching

Figure 10.2: Stimuli Developed for Testing Oral Form Recognition

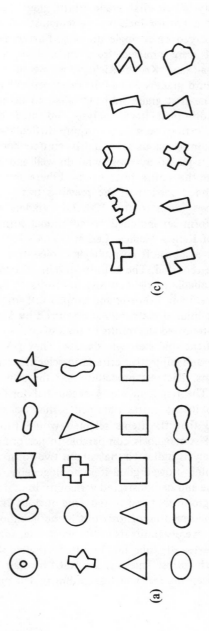

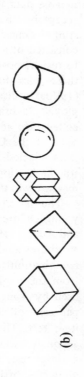

scores with the oral stereognosis score and found the visual task less difficult and only slightly related to the stereognosis scores.

Later, Arndt *et al.* (1970b) employed a slight procedural variation from that used previously. Their first grade, third grade, and adult subjects selected a visual match for each oral stereognostic form from five possible choices displayed on a single drawing. Furthermore, the three-dimensional stimuli were omitted from their form set. Test-retest, connected split half and Kruder-Richardson measures of test reliability revealed that third graders and adults produced satisfactorily reliable data. However, the first grade subjects failed to demonstrate acceptable reliability. Additional item analysis indicated that the stimuli ranged in difficulty from very easy to quite difficult and they consisted of a relatively homogeneous set. That is, an item contributes to test homogeneity if it is passed by those who do well and failed by those who do poorly on the entire test. Arndt, Elbert and Shelton (1970a) utilised an expanded version of the previous test which employed 35 oral stereognosis forms to test 100 third graders and 100 college age adults. This form set included 10 additional forms developed at the University of Kansas Medical Center (Figure 10.2c). Subjects selected the correct response from multiple choice drawings and standardisation data were reported. The authors determined that their measure was sufficiently reliable to yield consistent results.

The desirability of developing a shorter and simpler test for use with young children and brain-injured patients was discussed by McDonald and Aungst (1970). They reported the results of their efforts to develop an abbreviated version of the oral stereognosis task. They employed a combination of objective and subjective criteria in selecting ten forms from the original 25 items. The test procedure was the same as that used by Aungst (1965). The ten item scores accounted for 60 to 80 per cent of the variance in the scores obtained earlier using the 25 item test. This suggested that the items selected would provide an adequate measure of oral stereognosis comparable to performance on a longer test. An item analysis indicated that all but two forms were of moderate difficulty and nine showed good item homogeneity. The test was reported to be reliable and demonstrated variability in oral stereognosis for the limited age group that was tested. One obvious disadvantage of a short form of the oral stereognosis test is the likelihood of a reduced variability which severely limits its utility with older subjects.

The test procedures reviewed, thus far, required subjects to utilise the visual system to match forms. This was described by Lass, Tekieli and Eye (1971) as an intersensory task which according to data presented by Weinberg, Lyons and Liss (1970) provides a maturational advantage by the participation of the visual system. In an effort to develop a modality specific oral sensory task, Ringel, Burk and Scott (1970a) and Ringel *et al.* (1970b) devised an intrasensory form discrimination task. Their procedure required subjects to explore orally one form and then a second and report whether the two forms were the same or different. Their test employed ten forms (Figure 10.2a rows three and four) to construct 55 matching decisions. Each pair of forms was classified as either within the same geometric class (i.e. two triangles) or composed of different geometric classes. It was anticipated that this more discriminative assessment would more likely identify an oral sensory deficit in articulatory impaired subjects.

A number of investigators explored procedural variations applied to the same-different task. Lass *et al.* (1971) compared the performance of 30 normal-speaking college females on both the intersensory matching task, employing the 20 NIDR forms and the intrasensory form discrimination procedure employing 11 different forms. Their subjects achieved slightly, but significantly better scores on the intersensory matching task (73.6 per cent correct) than on the form discrimination (70.7 per cent correct). These findings support those of Ringel *et al.* (1970a). However, improved performance on the intersensory task was not confirmed by the work of Torrans and Beasley (1975). These authors administered a repeated measures design of the 10 forms used by Ringel *et al.* (1970a), the NIDR 20 set, the McDonald and Aungst (1970) abbreviated set, and the five three-dimensional form set to 40 normal adults. Each form set was administered to each subject as both an intersensory matching task and a form discrimination task. Two conditions were applied to each task: an unlimited exploration time and a five second time limit for studying the forms. The results indicated that the intersensory task was significantly more difficult than the form discrimination task.

The development of the form discrimination procedure raised the question of the role of retention of a sensory stimulus during the interval between the presentation of the second item of each stimulus pair. Lass and Clay (1973) addressed this issue in their study of children and college-age adults. They administered a repeated measures 11-form, 19-pair version of the Ringel procedure. Two conditions were employed: (1) simultaneous presentation of each form pair, and (2) sequential presentation (with a five second delay between each pair element). They observed no difference in performance for either group under the two conditions. However, Yairi and Cavaness (1975) administered the 55-pair Ringel task to two groups of young adults. One group received a simultaneous presentation condition and the other group was presented with one form at a time with a five second interval between forms. All subjects were allowed a seven second period orally to explore the forms. The authors reported significantly fewer errors were made under the successive than under the simultaneous condition.

The possible facilitative effect of learning on performance during multiple administrations of an oral form discrimination task was explored by Arndt *et al.* (1970a). They observed increased retest scores for both subject groups, suggesting a possible learning effect. Contradictory findings were evident in a series of studies reported by Lass *et al.* (1972). Each study employed the 10-form Ringel discrimination task administered to normal college-age subjects. The first study failed to show any improvement in the number of correct responses when subjects were informed of the accuracy of their discrimination than when they were not. In the second study subjects were retested four times at one week intervals. Again, no significant difference in subject performance was observed across the four administrations.

In addition to the number of oral stereognosis forms utilised in the various test versions and the various paradigms employed, several studies have explored variations in specific stimulus characteristics used to test oral form identification. Moser, LaGourgue and Class (1967) used six forms constructed in seven sizes and observed that correct form identifications increased with size but reached an asymptote at 0.25 in. Woodford (1964) explored the effects of variation in size, shape and thickness of forms. His results indicated that for all subjects manual discrimination was slightly superior than oral discrimination regardless of stimulus characteristics. Additional work on stimulus variables has been reported by Hochberg and Kabcenell (1967), Williams and LaPointe (1971) and Landt and Fransson (1975). While much work has been done on the comparison of intersensory matching with the intrasensory form discrimination procedure as well as numerous variations of number and type of stimuli employed, no report of standardisation data or item analyses has been published. Clearly psychometric principles remain to be applied to establish test reliability, item homogeneity and normative data.

Age and Oral Form Recognition

McDonald and Aungst (1967) employed the 25 item test to assess oral form recognition skill in subjects ranging from 6 years to 89 years. Subject performance showed improvement in mean score as a function of increasing age through mid-adolescence. Scores stabilised in the young adult range ($\overline{X}$ = 20.8) and a notable decrease in mean score was achieved by the geriatric subjects. The authors suggested that the levelling of the curve associated with the midteens may be related to completion of the growth of oral and facial structures. Furthermore, the decreased scores achieved by the elderly may represent an impairment or loss of efficiency in perceptual skills, or possibly an artifact of nursing home environment on perceptual performance. Similar findings concerning increased performance with age were reported by Arndt *et al.* (1970a, b) Ringel *et al.* (1970b) compared articulatory defective adults to normal-speaking children with a mean age of eight years. Ringel *et al.* (1970b) interpreted the higher adult scores as possibly due to their increased motor proficiency in manipulating the object or the increased ratio of oral cavity size to the size of the stimulus item. They also pointed out the possibility of other higher cortical advantages favouring the adult in a form discrimination task such as increased motivational levels, in addition to increased attention and retention spans. Additionally, Arndt *et al.* (1970b) suggested that increased test scores after the age of eight may relate to improved test-taking skills and learning effects. McDonald and Aungst (1970) administered ten oral stereognosis items to 200 elementary school children from kindergarten through third grade. Their results showed improved performance with age. It appears that the influence of age on oral form discrimination performance is one of the most consistent findings across studies in this area.

Subject Variables

Investigations of oral form recognition have explored a variety of subject variables including presence of articulation disorders, cleft palate, stuttering, brain injury, deafness, blindness and anaesthetisation. Interest in the relationship between articulatory defectiveness and oral form recognition developed as a logical extension of efforts to understand the control of the speech production mechanism. Moser *et al.* (1967) reported that stutterers and persons with articulation errors produced more error responses than normal subjects on an oral form identification task, while individuals with cerebral palsy made fewer correct responses than any of the other subject groups. Weinberg, Liss and Hillis (1970) tested visual, manual and oral form recognition in an articulatory defective and control group of junior and senior high students. Oral form recognition was the only statistically significant measure that distinguished the two groups. The work of Ringel *et al.* (1970a) observed a statistically significant difference between normal adults and those with articulation deficits. Similar findings were reported in studies of children by Ringel *et al.* (1970b), Fucci and Robertson (1971), Sommers, Cox and West (1972) and McNutt (1977). Evidence was reported by Arndt, Shelton, Johnson and Furr (1977) that oral form recognition was one of the few of the 45 measures which when subjected to a multivariate clustering procedure differentiated between subjects who misarticulated /r/ and /s/.

Several measures indirectly associated with articulatory competence have been explored in relation to oral form recognition. Locke (1968) reported that a group of normal subjects with high oral form recognition scores surpassed a normal group with low scores at a task that required learning to articulate foreign sounds. Madison and Fucci (1971) reported a correlation of —0.52 between scores on an oral form discrimination measure and The Wepman Auditory Discrimination Test, while Moreau and Lass (1974) found a significant but moderate correlation between a predictive articulation test and the form recognition test.

While the above evidence appears to support the thesis that deficits in oral form recognition may have some causal relationship to misarticulation, several studies provide contradictory evidence. McDonald and Aungst (1970) reported on the apparent independence of oral sensory function and articulatory proficiency. They cited the case of a spastic quadriplegic adult who had poor oral form recognition skills, poor oral two-point discrimination and an inability to sense his tongue position. His articulation, however, was described as within normal limits. Furthermore, they reported that there was essentially no relationship between oral stereognosis scores and ability to produce complex articulatory movements in 200 children from kindergarten through third grade. Admittedly, McDonald and Aungst (1970) employed the abbreviated test of oral form recognition which may have been insufficiently sensitive to document deficits in these children. Nevertheless, Baker in McDonald and Aungst (1970) reported similar findings for mentally retarded children. Additionally, Arndt *et al.* (1970a) failed to find a significant correlation between form recognition and articulation in a sample of physically normal children who made errors on the Templin-Darley Screening Articulation Test. Furthermore, LaPointe, Williams and Faircloth (1976) showed no relationship between oral form score and communicative ability in mentally retarded subjects.

If oral form identification skills do represent some measure of articulatory proficiency, then efforts to improve task performance should result in improvement in articulation and vice versa. Wilhelm (1971) taught subjects to match forms in an intersensory task which resulted in improved articulation while Shelton, Willis, Johnson and Arndt (1973) employed a similar oral training procedure with ten children and failed to observe an improvement in articulation. Ruscello (1972) administered two oral form identification tasks both before and after a period of speech therapy. Their subjects evidenced a small but statistically significant improvement on the oral form discrimination test.

Moser *et al.* (1967) reported data derived from several groups of subjects on a task similar to that used by McDonald and Aungst (1967). Blind subjects, deaf subjects with manual communication and deaf subjects with oral communication were compared with normals and performed similarly on a task of oral form identification. Additionally, the authors observed no correlation between intelligence and oral form perception. In contrast to the previous findings, Bishop, Ringel and House (1972) compared deaf speakers and normal subjects on measures of two-point discrimination, as well as manual and oral form discrimination. Performance on the oral form discrimination task was the only measure which distinguished the groups. In a second study by the same group of authors (Bishop *et al.*, 1973) manually deaf communicators were inferior to orally educated deaf and normal subjects, while the latter two groups were similar in their performance on an oral form discrimination measure.

Similar contradictory evidence exists regarding cleft-palate subjects and oral form recognition ability. Mason (1967) and Catalanotto and Moss (1973) found no difference between cleft palate persons and normals on a task of oral form recognition, while studies by Hochberg and Kabcenell (1967), Andrews (1973) and Pressel and Hochberg (1974) did report differences. Problems of comparability of these studies in terms of subject characteristics and variability prompted Pressel and Hochberg (1974) to state that they were unable to conclude that children with cleft palate differ from normals with respect to their oral form discrimination ability.

Several studies have explored oral sensory functioning in the adult brain-injured population. Levine (1965) observed that aphasic subjects made significantly more errors (approximately three times as many) on a test of oral form recognition than did normals. Identification of an associated oral sensory deficit in the speech apraxic population has been the subject of several investigations (Guilford and Hawk, 1968;

Rosenbek *et al.*, 1973; Teixeira, Defran and Nichols, 1974). Results of these studies have indicated that as a group, speech apraxic subjects produced more error responses on an oral stereognosis task than did aphasic, dysarthric or normal control populations. These findings have been interpreted to reflect a deficit in cortical sensory functioning; consequently, they challenge the traditional limited view that speech apraxia is the exclusive result of disrupted motor speech control. The actual contribution of oral stereognostic perceptual problems to accurate articulatory control in brain-injured subjects remains questionable in view of the heterogeneity of the observed deficit in this population. Specifically, Rosenbek *et al.* (1973) 'observed that less than half of their apraxic subjects scored outside the range of errors for the normal and aphasic groups' (p. 27). Furthermore, data from Teixeira *et al.* (1974) indicated that half of their apraxic subjects scored within the error range achieved by the aphasics. Thus, it is evident that the speech apraxic subjects studied have failed to display a uniform deficit.

Site of cortical lesion and an oral stereognostic deficit was explored by Baxter, Simpson, Greenbaum and Pribram (1980). They reported a moderate correlation between task performance and a posterior lesion. In contrast, Deutsch (1981) reported that despite the traditional association of a cortical sensory deficit including astereognosis in posterior brain-injured patients, oral form identification scores failed to differ significantly for anterior and posterior brain-lesioned subjects exhibiting speech apraxic behaviours and aphasia. In addition, when the total group performance was compared to data of previous studies, apraxics exhibited a deficit in oral form identification ability when compared to normals, but they appeared to perform similarly to aphasic subjects in other studies. Furthermore, performance on the oral form identification task was shown to be unrelated to speech production severity measures. Results were interpreted to suggest that oral form identification deficits are most probably not causally related to motor speech programming problems but rather indicate some degree of relationship with impaired discrimination of linguistic symbols as a consequence of a larger aphasic involvement.

Oral form identification has been investigated in several other populations. Edentulous patients performed comparably with and without their dentures on tasks that involved variation in size, shape, and thickness of forms (Woodford, 1964). This supports McDonald and Aungst's (1967) report that normals exhibited no difference in the mean number of correct form identifications when the palate was covered with dental wax or uncovered. These results most probably relate to the general findings of several studies which have tested various parameters of oral sensitivity and have demonstrated that the oral region does not possess a uniform sensitivity in response to stimulation. Specifically, Ringel (1970) stated that 'oral form recognition is a skill for which lingual sensitivity and manipulation are paramount' and 'the progression from maximal to minimal discrimination involves lingual, labial and palatal structures, in that order' (p. 196). Studies involving subjects who have undergone nerve block anaesthetisation are open to various interpretations because of the likelihood that motor nerves and responses of the central nervous system may also be affected by the drug. Ringel (1970) has reviewed various controversies associated with these oral anaesthetisation studies.

Unfortunately, despite much of the preliminary work which was directed toward standardisation of the oral stereognosis task, considerable effort has been expended on the development of numerous test variations employing different numbers of forms and a variety of stimulus modifications each administered to subjects with different types of communicative impairments. Results of these studies have provided some insights concerning a number of relevant variables. However, it is difficult to make comparative statements across studies because of the different procedural, stimulus, and subject variables employed.

Conclusion

From the preceding review of the literature, it is apparent that oral stereognosis testing has failed to document a consistent deficit among speech-disordered populations. This raises the question of the validity of the task. Specifically, is oral form identification a true measure of oral sensory function? While there is little disagreement that oral form identification does involve some parameter(s) of oral sensation, it is likely that it also incorporates such additional skills as retention, cognitive processing, verbal mediation abilities, anatomical maturation and motor skills.

Keslinger (1973) pointed out that the validity of behavioural or cognitive measures is often difficult to determine and he discussed three ways to establish validity of a test or measurement. When these are related to oral form identification some rather obvious limitations of the task as an index of oral sensory perception become apparent. First, the establishment of content validity requires identification of all behaviours which constitute oral sensory perception. While considerable progress has been made in histological and electrophysiological investigations, the present state of our knowledge concerning oral sensory perception remains incomplete. Thus, we are unable to achieve this requirement. Second, criterion validity is the degree to which oral form identification correlates with known indicators of oral sensory integrity. Neither concurrent nor predictive criterion validity has been consistently documented in studies attempting to correlate oral form identification with articulatory defectiveness. The third approach relates to construct validity. This reflects the degree to which oral form identification confirms some theoretical construct or explanation of oral sensory function. Construct validity is verified if measurements agree with theoretical predictions, but failure to verify the prediction may be a result of either an invalid measure or an incorrect theory or both. Clearly the McDonald and Aungst (1970) report of a cerebral palsy patient who spoke with normal articulation but exhibited poor oral form recognition skill, poor oral two-point discrimination and inability to sense tongue position, questions the construct validity of present measures of oral sensory function related to speech production.

Certainly much knowledge has been gained in our understanding of somaesthesis and the role of sensory mechanisms in speech production. However, the 'assessment of oral somestheses has found no secure place in the practice of speech pathology' (Shelton, 1979: p. 140). The present evidence argues against a simple causal relationship between reduced oral sensory abilities and speech disorders. Clearly, the tasks we use to measure oral discrimination abilities will require further study, refinement and standardisation. It is anticipated that pursuit of neurophysiological parameters of oral somaesthesis will provide greater understanding of the sensory systems underlying speech production without the complexities inherent in the behavioural measurement of perception. In the interim, evidence supporting the view that normal speech production in some manner utilises oral sensation persists and the practising speech pathologist would do well to continue to employ a multimodality stimulation approach in remediation of the articulatory-impaired patient.

REFERENCES

Aaronson, D. (1967) 'Temporal Factors in Perception and Short Term Memory', *Psychological Bulletin*, *67*, 130-44.

Aaronson, D., Markowitz, N. and Shapiro, H. (1971) 'Perception and Immediate Recall of Normal and Compressed Auditory Sequences', *Perception and Psychophysics*, *9*, 344-88.

Abberton, E. (1976) 'A Laryngographic Study of Voice Quality', unpublished PhD thesis, University of London.

Abberton, E., Ashby, M.G. and Fourcin, A.J. (1976) 'Speech Patterns in the Teaching of Pronunciation' in Lindblom, B. and Nordstrom, P.E. (eds.), *Fonetik och Uttalspedagogik*, University of Stockholm.

Abberton, E. and Fourcin, A.J. (1972) 'Laryngographic Analysis and Intonation', *British Journal of Disorders of Communication*, *7*, 24-9.

Abberton, E. and Fourcin, A.J. (1975) 'Visual Feedback and the Acquisition of Intonation' in Lenneberg, E. and Lenneberg, E. (eds.), *Foundations of Language Development, a Multi-disciplinary Approach*, Vol. *2*, Academic Press, New York, p. 10.

Abberton, E. and Fourcin, A.J. (1978) 'Intonation and Speaker Identification', *Language and Speech*, *21*, 305-18.

Abberton, E., Parker, A. and Fourcin, A.J. (1977) 'Speech Improvement in Deaf Adults using Laryngograph Displays', *Papers from the Research Conference on Speech Analysing Aids for the Deaf*, Gallaudet College, Washington, D.C.

Agnello, J.G. (1975) 'Measurements and Analysis of Visible Speech' in Singh, S. (ed.), *Measurement Procedures in Speech, Hearing and Language*, University Park Press, Baltimore.

Albert, M. and Bear, D. (1974) 'Time to Understand: a Case Study of Word Deafness with Reference to the Role of Time in Auditory Comprehension', *Brain*, *97*, 196-208.

Allen, J. (1980) 'Hemispherical Specialization in Stuttering', paper presented at the Institute of Acoustics Speech Group Meeting: Speech Production and Perception in the Disabled, London, February.

Andrews, J.R. (1973) 'Oral Form Discrimination in Individuals with Normal and Cleft Palates', *Cleft Palate Journal*, *10*, 92-8.

Angelocci, A.A., Kopp, G.A. and Holbrook, A. (1964) 'The Vowel

Formants of Deaf and Normal-hearing Eleven-to-fourteen-year-old Boys', *Journal of Speech and Hearing Disorders*, *29*, 156-70.

Anthony, J. (1978) 'The Voiscope', *Health Services Bulletin, Scottish Home and Health Department*, *36*, 321-8.

Anthony, J. (1980) 'Aerodynamic and Phonetic Analysis' in Edwards, M. and Watson, A.C.H. (eds.), *Advances in the Management of Cleft Palate*, Churchill-Livingstone, Edinburgh.

Anthony, J. and MacLachlan, D. (1969) 'A Small Transducer for sub-glottal pressure measurement', *Work in Progress, 3, Department of Linguistics, University of Edinburgh*.

Ardran, G.M. and Kemp, F.H. (1967) 'Laryngeal Function Following Lateral Fixation of the Vocal Cord', *British Journal of Disorders of Communication*, *2*, 15-22.

Arndt, W.B., Elbert, M. and Shelton, R.L. (1970a) 'Standardization of a Test of Oral Stereognosis', in Bosma, J.F. (ed.), *Second Symposium on Oral Sensation and Perception*, Charles C. Thomas, Springfield, Ill.

Arndt, W.B., Gauer, J., Shelton, R.L., Crary, D. and Chisum, L. (1970b) 'Refinement of a Test of Oral Stereognosis' in Bosma, J.F. (ed.), *Second Symposium on Oral Sensation and Perception*, Charles C. Thomas, Springfield, Ill.

Arndt, W.B., Shelton, R.L., Johnson, A.F. and Furr, M.L. (1977) 'Identification and Description of Homogeneous Subgroups Within a Sample of Misarticulating Children', *Journal of Speech and Hearing Research*, *20*, 263-92.

Arnott, G., Lhote-Munier, E., Vaneclou, F. and Milbled, G. (1975) 'Sonographic and Auditory Analysis of Dysarthria in a Case of Steele-Olaewski-Richardson Syndrome', *Folia Phoniatrica, 27*, 443-56.

Aungst, L.F. (1965) 'The Relationship Between Oral Stereognosis and Articulation Proficiency', unpublished Doctoral thesis, Pennsylvania State University.

Baer, T., Gay, T. and Niimi, S. (1976) 'Control of Fundamental Frequency, Intensity and Register of Phonation', *Haskins Laboratories Status Report on Speech Research*, SR-45/46, 175-85.

Balasubramanian, T. (1981) 'The Pure Oral Vowels of Colloquial Tamil – an x-ray Photographic Study', *Journal of the International Phonetic Association*, *11*, 27-34.

Ball, M.J. (1976) 'Towards a Description of the North Welsh Monophthongs', unpublished MA thesis, University of Essex.

Bar, A., Singer, J. and Feldman, R.G. (1969) 'Subvocal Muscle Activity During Stuttering and Fluent Speech: a Comparison', *Journal of the South African Logopedic Society, 16*, 14-19.

Basmajian, J.V. (1978) *Muscles Alive*, Williams and Wilkins, Baltimore.

Basmajian, J.V. (1981) 'Biofeedback in Rehabilitation: a Review of Principles and Practices', *Archives of Physical Medicine and Rehabilitation, 62*, 469-75.

Baxter, S., Simpson, M., Greenbaum, H. and Pribram, H. (1980) 'Localization of Phonological Realization Disorders in Aphasia with Three-Dimensional Computerised Tomography', paper presented at Academy of Aphasia, South Yarmouth, Mass.

Beasley, D.S. and Beasley, D.C. (1973) 'Auditory Reassembly Abilities of Black and White First- and Third Grade Children', *Journal of Speech and Hearing Research, 16*, 213-21.

Beasley, D.S., Bratt, G.W. and Rintelmann, W.F. (1980) 'Intelligibility of Time-compressed Sentential Stimuli', *Journal of Speech and Hearing Research, 23*, 722-31.

Beasley, D.S. and Flaherty-Rintelmann, A. (1976) 'Children's Perception of Temporally Distorted Sentential Approximations of Varying Length', *Audiology, 15*, 315-25.

Beasley, D.S., Forman, B.S. and Rintelmann, W.F. (1972a) 'Perception of Time-compressed CNC Monosyllables', *Journal of Auditory Research, 12*, 71-5.

Beasley, D.S. and Freeman, B.A. (1977) 'Time-altered Speech as a Measure of Central Auditory Processing' in Keith, R. (ed.), *Central Auditory Dysfunction*, Grune and Stratton, London.

Beasley, D.S. and Maki, J.E. (1976) 'Time- and Frequency-altered Speech' in Lass, N.J. (ed.), *Contemporary Issues in Experimental Phonetics,* Academic Press, New York.

Beasley, D.S., Maki, J.E. and Orchik, D.J. (1976) 'Children's Perception of Time-compressed Speech Using Two Measures of Speech Discrimination', *Journal of Speech and Hearing Disorders, 41*, 216-25.

Beasley, D.S., Schwimmer, S. and Rintelmann, W.F. (1972b) 'Intelligibility of Time-compressed CNC Monosyllables', *Journal of Speech and Hearing Research, 15*, 340-50.

Beasley, D.S. and Shriner, T.H. (1973) 'Auditory Analysis of Temporally Distorted Sentential Approximations', *Audiology: Journal of Auditory Communication, 12*, 262-71.

Beasley, D.S., Shriner, T.H., Manning, W.H. and Beasley, D.C. (1974) 'Auditory Assembly of CVC's by Children with Normal and Defective Articulation', *Journal of Communication Disorders, 7*, 127-33.

Beaumont, G.J. and Rugg, M.D. (1978) 'Neuropsychological Laterality of Function and Dyslexia', *Dyslexia Review*, *1*, 18-21.

Beaumont, J.T. and Foss, B.M. (1957) 'Individual Differences in Reacting to Delayed Auditory Feedback', *British Journal of Psychology*, *48*, 85-9.

Bergstrom, L.V. (1978) 'Congenital and Acquired Deafness in Clefting and Craniofacial Syndromes', *Cleft Palate Journal*, *15*, 254-61.

Berlin, C.I. and Cullen, J.K. Jnr. (1977) 'Acoustic Problems in Dichotic Listening Tasks' in Segalowitz, S.J. and Gruber, F.G. (eds.), *Language Development and Neurological Theory*, Academic Press, New York.

Berlin, C.I. and McNeil, M.R. (1976) 'Dichotic Listening' in Lass, N.J. (ed.), *Contemporary Issues in Experimental Phonetics*, Academic Press, New York.

Berry, M.F. and Eisenson, J. (1957) *Speech Disorders*, Appleton Century Crofts, New York.

Berry, R.J., Epstein, R., Fourcin, A.J., Freeman, M., MacCurtain, F. and Noscoe, N. (1982a) 'An Objective Analysis of Voice Disorder: Part One', *British Journal of Disorders of Communication*, *17*, 67-76.

Berry, R.J., Epstein, R., Freeman, M., MacCurtain, F. and Noscoe, N. (1982b) 'An Objective Analysis of Voice Disorder: Part Two', *British Journal of Disorders of Communication*, *17*, 77-85.

Bishop, M.E., Ringel, R.L. and House, A.S. (1972) 'Orosensory Perception in the Deaf', *Volta Review*, *74*, 289-98.

Bishop, M.E., Ringel, R.L. and House, A.S. (1973) 'Orosensory Perception, Speech Production and Deafness', *Journal of Speech and Hearing Research*, *16*, 257-66.

Bladon, R.A.W. and Nolan, F.J. (1977) 'A Video-fluorographic Investigation of Tip and Blade Alveolars in English', *Journal of Phonetics*, *5*, 185-93.

Blanchard, S.L. and Prescott, T.E. (1980) 'The Effects of Temporal Expansion upon Auditory Comprehension in Aphasic Adults', *British Journal of Disorders of Communication*, *15*, 115-27.

Blom, S. (1960) 'Afferent Influences on Tongue Muscle Activity', *Acta Physiologica Scandinavia*, *49* Suppl. 170, 1-97.

Bloodstein, O. (1979) *Speech Pathology: An Introduction*, Houghton and Mifflin, Boston.

Blumstein, S.E., Cooper, W.E., Goodglass, H., Statlender, S. and Gottlieb, J. (1980) 'Production Deficits in Aphasia: A Voice-Onset-Time Analysis', *Brain and Language*, *9*, 153-70.

Blumstein, S.E., Cooper, W.E., Zurif, E.B. and Caramazza, A. (1977) 'The Perception and Production of Voice Onset Time in Aphasia', *Neuropsychologia*, *15*, 371-83.

Blumstein, S., Goodglass, H. and Tartter, V. (1975) 'The Reliability of Ear Advantage in Dichotic Listening', *Brain and Language*, *2*, 226-36.

Bocca, E. and Calearo, C. (1963) 'Central Hearing Processes' in Jerger, J. (ed.), *Modern Developments in Audiology*, Academic Press, New York.

Boller, F. and Marcie, P. (1978) 'Possible Role of Abnormal Auditory Feedback in Conduction Aphasia', *Neuropsychologia*, *16*, 521-4.

Boller, F., Vrtunski, P.B., Kim, Y. and Mack, J.L. (1978) 'Delayed Auditory Feedback and Aphasia', *Cortex*, *14*, 212-26.

Bond, Z.S. and Wilson, H.F. (1980) 'Acquisition of the Voicing Contrast by Language Delayed and Normal-Speaking Children', *Journal of Speech and Hearing Research*, *23*, 152-61.

Borden, G.J. (1979) 'An Interpretation of Research on Feedback Interruption in Speech', *Brain and Language*, *7*, 307-19.

Borden, G.J., Dorman, M.F., Freeman, F.J. and Niimi, S. (1976) 'Coordination of Phonation and Articulation During Delayed Auditory Feedback', paper presented at the American Speech and Hearing Association Convention, Houston, Texas.

Borden, G.J. and Harris, K.S. (1980) *Speech Science Primer: Physiology, Acoustics and Perception of Speech*, Williams and Wilkins, Baltimore.

Bordley, J. and Haskins, J. (1955) 'The Role of the Cerebrum in Hearing', *Annals of Otology, Rhinology, and Laryngology, 64*, 370-82.

Bosma, J.F. (ed.) (1967) *Symposium on Oral Sensation and Perception*, Charles C. Thomas, Springfield, Ill.

Bosma, J.F. (ed.) (1970) *Second Symposium on Oral Sensation and Perception*, Charles C. Thomas, Springfield, Ill.

Bouhuys, A., Proctor, D.F. and Mead, J. (1966) 'Kinetic Aspects of Singing', *Journal of Applied Psychology*, *21*, 483-96.

Bowman, J.P., Jr. (1971) *The Muscle Spindle and Neural Control of the Tongue: Implications for Speech*, Charles C. Thomas, Springfield, Ill.

Bowman, S.A. and Shanks, J.C. (1978) 'Velopharyngeal Relationships of /i/ and /s/ as Seen Cephalometrically for Persons with Suspected Incompetence', *Journal of Speech and Hearing Disorders*, *43*, 185-91.

Boyd, I.A., Eyzaguirre, C., Matthews, P.B.C. and Rushworth, G. (1968)

The Role of the Gamma System in Movement and Posture, Association for the Aid of Crippled Children, New York.

Boyd, I.A. and Rcberts, T.D.M. (1953) 'Proprioceptive Discharges from Stretch Receptors in the Knee Joint of the Cat', *Journal of Physiology*, *122*, 38-58.

Brady, J.P. and Berson, J. (1975) 'Stuttering, Dichotic Listening and Cerebral Dominance', *Archives of General Psychiatry*, *32*, 1449-52.

Brady, W.A. (1978) 'Auditory and Visual Response Patterns of Right and Left Tempero-parietal Lobe Damaged Patients for Linguistic and Non-linguistic Dichotic Stimuli', unpublished PhD thesis, Kent State University, Ohio.

Brayton, E.R. and Conture, E.G. (1978) 'Effects of Noise and Rhythmic Stimulation on the Speech of Stutterers', *Journal of Speech and Hearing Research*, *21*, 285-94.

Brazil, D. (1975) *Discourse Intonation*, Birmingham University Discourse Analysis Monographs, *1*.

Broadbent, D. (1954) 'The Role of Auditory Localization in Attention and Memory', *Journal of Experimental Psychology*, *47*, 191-6.

Brodnitz, F.S. (1965) *Vocal Rehabilitation*, American Academy of Ophthamology and Otolaryngology, New York.

Brookshire, R.H. (1973) *An Introduction to Aphasia*, BRK Publishers, Minneapolis.

Brown, J.W. (1975) 'On the Neural Organization of Language: Thalmic and Cortical Relationships', *Brain and Language*, *2*, 18-30.

Brown, J.W. (1978) 'Lateralization: a Brain Model', *Brain and Language*, *5*, 258-61.

Brown, J.W. (1979) 'Language Representation in the Brain' in Steklis, H.D. and Raleigh, M.J. (eds.), *Neurobiology of Social Communication in Primates*, Academic Press, New York.

Bryden, M.P. (1963) 'Ear Preference in Auditory Perception', *Journal of Experimental Psychology*, *65*, 103-5.

Bryden, M.P. and Allard, F. (1978) 'Dichotic Listening and the Development of Linguistic Processes' in Kinsbourne, M. (ed.), *Asymmetrical Function of the Brain*, Cambridge University Press, Cambridge.

Bryden, M.P., Ley, G. and Sugarman, J.H. (1982) 'A Left-ear Advantage for Identifying the Emotional Quality of Tonal Sequences', *Neuropsychologia*, *20*, 83-7.

Buffery, A.W. and Burton, A. (1982) 'Information Processing and Redevelopment: Towards a Science of Neuropsychological Rehabilitation' in Burton, A. (ed.), *The Pathology and Psychology of*

Cognition, Methuen, London.

Burgess, P.R. and Clark, R.J. (1969) 'Characteristics of Knee Joint Receptors in the Cat', *Journal of Physiology*, *203*, 317-35.

Butler, R.A. and Galloway, F.T. (1957) 'Factoral Analysis of the Delayed Auditory Feedback Phenomenon', *Journal of the Acoustical Society of America*, *29*, 632-5.

Buxton, L.F. (1969) 'An Investigation of Sex and Age Differences in Speech Behaviour under Delayed Auditory Feedback', unpublished PhD thesis, Ohio State University.

Calearo, C. and Lazzaroni, A. (1957) 'Speech Intelligibility in Relation to the Speed of Message', *Laryngoscope*, *67*, 410-9.

Calearo, C., Teatini, G. and Pestalozza, G. (1962) 'Speech Intelligibility in the Presence of Interrupted Noise', *Journal of Auditory Research*, *2*, 179-86.

Camougis, G. (1970) *Nerves, Muscles and Electricity*, Appleton-Century-Crofts, New York.

Carpenter, R. and Rutherford, D. (1973) 'Acoustic Cue Discrimination in Adult Aphasia', *Journal of Speech and Hearing Research*, *16*, 534-44.

Castro-Caldas, A. and Botelho, M.A.S. (1980) 'Dichotic Listening in the Recovery of Aphasia after Stroke', *Brain and Language*, *10*, 145-51.

Catalanotto, F.A. and Moss, J.L. (1973) 'Manual and Oral Stereognosis in Children with Cleft Palate, Gonadal Dysgenesis, Pseudohypoparathryoidism, Oral Facial Digital Syndrome, and Kallman's Syndrome', *Archives of Oral Biology*, *48*, 1227-32.

Cermak, L.S. and Moreines, J. (1976) 'Verbal Retention Deficits in Aphasic and Amnesic Patients', *Brain and Language*, *3*, 16-27.

Chapin, C., Blumstein, S.E., Meisser, B. and Boller, F. (1981) 'Speech Production Mechanisms in Aphasia: a Delayed Auditory Feedback Study', *Brain and Language*, *14*, 106-13.

Chase, R.A., Sutton, S., First, D. and Zubin, J. (1961) 'A Developmental Study of Changes in Behavior under Delayed Auditory Feedback', *Journal of Genetic Psychology*, *99*, 101-12.

Chasty, H. (1979) 'Functional Asymmetry of the Brain in Normal Children and Dyslexics', *Dyslexia Review*, *2*, 9-12.

Chasty, H. (1981) 'Dichotic Stimulation Effects in Dyslexics and Normal Children', *Dyslexia Review*, *4*, 8-9.

Cherry, C. and Sayer, B. (1956) 'Experiments upon the Total Inhibition of Stammering by External Control and Some Clinical Results', *Journal of Psychosomatic Research*, *1*, 233-46.

Christensen, J.M., Weinberg, G. and Alfonso, P.J. (1978) 'Productive

Voice Onset Time Characteristics of Esophogeal Speech', *Journal of Speech and Hearing Research*, *21*, 56-62.

Chusid, J.G. (1973) *Correlative Neuroanatomy and Functional Neurology*, Lange Medical Publications, Los Altos, CA.

Clark, R.G. (1975) *Manter and Gatz's Essentials of Clinical Neuroanatomy and Neurophysiology*, 5th edn, F.A. Davis Co., Philadephia, PA.

Clasquin, M. (1980) 'Recall of Word Sequences as a Function of Time Compression and Grammaticality by Older Adults', unpublished MA thesis, Memphis State University, Tennessee.

Code, C. (1979) 'Genuine and Artificial Stammering: an EMG Comparison', *British Journal of Disorders of Communication*, *14*. 5-16.

Code, C. (1980) 'Delayed Auditory Feedback and Auditory Feedback Masking with Stammerers and Normal Speakers', *Australian Journal of Human Communication Disorders, 8,* 40-8.

Code, C. (1981) 'Dichotic Listening with the Communicatively Impaired: Results from Trials of a Short British-English Dichotic Word Test', *Journal of Phonetics*, *9*, 375-83.

Code, C. (1982) 'Neurolinguistic Analysis of Recurrent Utterances in Aphasia', *Cortex*, *18*, 141-52.

Code, C. (1983a) 'The Validity of Dichotic Listening as an Indicator of Hemispheric Shift in Aphasia: Dominance vs. Lesion Effects in the Performance of Fluent and Non Fluent Subjects', paper presented at Dysphasia Conference, Middlesex Hospital, London.

Code, C. (1983b) 'Hemispheric Specialization Retraining in Aphasia: Possibilities and Problems' in Code, C. and Muller, D.J. (eds.), *Aphasia Therapy*, Edward Arnold, London.

Code, C. and Ball, M.J. (1982) 'Fricative Production in Broca's Aphasia: a Spectrographic Analysis', *Journal of Phonetics*, *10*, 325-31.

Colcord, R.D. and Adams, M.R. (1979) 'Voicing Duration and Vocal SPL Changes Associated with Stuttering Reduction During Singing', *Journal of Speech and Hearing Research*, *22*, 468-79.

Collins, M., Rosenbek, J.C. and Wertz, R.T. (1978) 'Spectrographic Analysis of Vowel and Word Duration in Apraxia of Speech', paper presented at the American Speech and Hearing Association Convention, San Francisco, California.

Cooper, F.S. (1965) 'Research Techniques and Instrumentation: EMG' in *Proceedings of the Conferences: Communicative Problems in Cleft Palate, ASHA Reports, 1,* 153-68.

Cooper, M. (1974) 'Spectrographic Analysis of Fundamental Frequency and Hoarseness Before and After Vocal Rehabilitation', *Journal of Speech and Hearing Disorders*, *34*, 286-97.

Cooper, R., Osselton, J.W. and Shaw, J.C. (1974) *EEG Technology*, Butterworths, London.

Cooper, S. (1953) 'Muscle Spindles in the Intrinsic Muscles of the Tongue', *Journal of Physiology*, *122*, 193-202.

Critchley, M. (1953) *The Parietal Lobes*, Edward Arnold, London.

Crosson, R. and Warren, R.L. (1981) 'Dichotic Ear Preferences for C-V-C Words in Wernicke's and Broca's Aphasia', *Cortex*, *17*, 249-58.

Crystal, D. (1975) *The English Tone of Voice*, Edward Arnold, London.

Curlee, R.F. and Perkins, W.H. (1969) 'Conversational Rate Control Therapy for Stuttering', *Journal of Speech and Hearing Disorders*, *34*, 245-50.

Curry, F.K.W. (1967) 'A Comparison of Left Handed and Right Handed Subjects on Verbal and Non-verbal Dichotic Listening Tasks', *Cortex*, *3*, 343-52.

Curry, F.K.W. and Gregory, H.H. (1969) 'The Performance of Stutterers on Dichotic Listening Tasks Thought to Reflect Cerebral Dominance', *Journal of Speech and Hearing Research*, *12*, 73-82.

Damasio, H. and Damasio, A.R. (1979) '"Paradoxic" Extinction in Dichotic Listening: Possible Anatomic Significance', *Neurology*, *29*, 644-53.

Daniloff, R.G., Shriner, T.H. and Zemlin, W.R. (1968) 'Intelligibility of Vowels Altered in Duration and Frequency', *Journal of the Acoustical Society of America*, *44*, 700-7.

Darley, F.L., Aronson, A.E. and Brown, J.R. (1975) *Motor Speech Disorders*, W.B. Saunders, Philadelphia.

Darwin, C.J. (1971) 'Ear Differences in the Recall of Fricatives and Vowels', *Quarterly Journal of Experimental Psychology*, *23*, 46-62.

Darwin, C.J. (1974) 'Ear Differences and Hemispheric Specialization' in Schmidt, F.O. and Worden, F. (eds.), *The Neurosciences*, vol. 3, MIT Press, Cambridge, Massachusetts.

Davis, J.F. (1952) *Manual of Surface Electromyography*, Laboratory for Psychological Studies, Allan Memorial Institute of Psychiatry, Montreal.

De Chicchis, A., Orchik, D.J. and Tecca, J. (1981) 'The Effect of Word List and Talker Variation on Word Recognition Scores Using Time-altered Speech', *Journal of Speech and Hearing Disorders*, *46*, 213-6.

Delattre, P. (1962) 'Some Factors of Vowel Duration and Their Cross-linguistic Validity', *Journal of the Acoustical Society of America*, *34*, 1141-2.

Delattre, P., Liberman, A.M. and Cooper, F.S. (1955) 'Acoustic Loci and Transitional Cues for Consonants', *Journal of the Acoustical Society of America, 27*, 769-73.

De Quiros, J. (1964) 'Accelerated Speech Audiometry, and Examination of Test Results' translated by Tonndorf, J. (ed.), *Translations of the Beltone Institute of Hearing Research, No. 17*, Chicago.

De Santis, M., Cellini, N., Minuto, I., Modica, V. and Ciarniello, V. (1979) 'Xeroradiography, Teleradiography at High Voltage, Opaque Contrastography in the Dynamic Study of the Cervical Portion of Esophagus in Patients who are [sic] Undergone Laryngectomy and Radiotherapy', *Acta Medica Romana, 17*, 255-9.

Deutsch, S.E. (1981) 'Oral Form Identification as a Measure of Cortical Sensory Dysfunction in Apraxia of Speech and Aphasia', *Journal of Communication Disorders, 14*, 65-73.

Dewar, A., Dewar, A.D. and Anthony, J.F.K. (1976) 'The Effect of Auditory Feedback Masking on Concomitant Movements of Stammering', *British Journal of Disorders of Communication, 11*, 95-102.

Dicenta, M. and Oliveras, J. (1976) 'La Xerorradiología Laríngea', *Acta Otorrinolaringologica Española, 27*, 99-106.

Doran, P. and Riensche, L. (1981) 'Stutterers and Nonstutterers Central Auditory Abilities as Measured by Time-compressed Speech', paper presented at the Mid-South Conference on Communicative Disorders, Memphis, Tennessee.

Dorman, M.F. and Porter, R.J. (1975) 'Hemispheric Lateralization for Speech Perception in Stutterers', *Cortex, 11*, 181-5.

Downie, A.W., Low, J.M. and Lindsay, D.D. (1981) 'Speech Disorder in Parkinsonism: Usefulness of Delayed Auditory Feedback in Selected Cases', *British Journal of Disorders of Communication, 16*, 135-9.

Draper, M.H., Ladefoged, P. and Whitteridge, D. (1960) 'Expiratory Pressures and Airflow During Speech', *British Medical Journal, 264*, 1837-43.

Duchenne, G.B.A. (1949) *Physiologie des Mouvements* (1867), translated by E.B. Kaplan, W.B. Saunders, Philadelphia.

Ebbin, J. and Edwards, A. (1967) 'Speech Sound Discrimination when Inter-sound Interval is Varied', *Journal of Speech and Hearing Research, 10*, 120-5.

Echols-Chambers, L. (1981) 'Low Frequency Hearing Impairment in Presbycusis: Implicant of Central Aging?', unpublished M.A. thesis, Purdue University, West Lafayette, Indiana.

Efron, R. (1963) 'Temporal Perception, Aphasia, and Deja Vu', *Brain, 86*, 403-24.

Eguchi, S. and Hirsh, I. (1969) 'Development of Speech Sounds in Children', *Acta Otolaryngology Supplement*, 257.

Ellis, R.E. (1979) 'The Exeter Nasal Anemometry System' in Ellis, R.E. and Flack, F.C. (eds.), *Diagnosis and Treatment of Palato Glossal Malfunction*, The College of Speech Therapists, London.

Ellis, R.E., Flack, F.C., Curle, H.J. and Selley, W.G. (1978) 'A System for the Assessment of Nasal Airflow During Speech', *British Journal of Disorders of Communication*, *13*, 31-40.

Emerick, L.L. and Hatten, J.T. (1974) *Diagnosis and Evaluation in Speech Pathology*, Prentice-Hall, Englewood Cliffs, N.J.

Enany, N.M. (1981) 'A Cephalometric Study of the Effects of Primary Osteoplasty in Unilateral Cleft Lip and Palate Individuals', *Cleft Palate Journal*, *18*, 286-92.

Faaberg-Andersen, K.L. (1957) 'Electromyographic Investigation of Intrinsic Muscles in Humans: an Investigation of Subjects with Normally Movable Vocal Cords and Patients with Vocal Cord Paresis', *Acta Physiology Scandinavia*, *41*, suppl. 140, 1-148.

Faaberg-Andersen, K.L. (1964) 'Electromyography of the Laryngeal Muscles in Man' in Brewer, D.W. (ed.), *Research Potentials in Voice Physiology (International Conference 1961)*. State University of New York Press, New York, 105-29.

Fabre, P. (1957) 'Un Procédé Electrique Percutané d'Inscription de l'Accolement Glottique au Cours de la Phonation: Glottographie de Haute Fréquence. Premiers Résultats', *Bull. Acad. Nat. Méd.*, *141*, 69-99.

Fairbanks, G. (1954) 'A Theory of the Speech Mechanism as a Servo-System', Reproduced in *Experimental Phonetics: Selected Articles by Grant Fairbanks* (1966), University of Illinois Press, Illinois.

Fairbanks, G. (1955) 'Selective Vocal Effects of Delayed Auditory Feedback Upon Articulation', Reproduced in *Experimental Phonetics: Selected Articles by Grant Fairbanks* (1966), University of Illinois Press, Illinois.

Fairbanks, G., Everitt, W.L. and Jaeger, R.P. (1954) 'Methods for Time or Frequency Compression-expansion of Speech', *Transactions of I.R.E. – P.G.A. AU*-2, 7-12.

Fairbanks, G., Guttman, N. and Miron, M.S. (1957) 'Auditory Comprehension of Repeated High-speed Messages', *Journal of Speech and Hearing Disorders*, *22*, 20-22.

Fairbanks, G. and Kodman, F. (1957) 'Word Intelligibility as a Function of Time-compression', *Journal of the Acoustical Society of America*, *29*, 636-41.

Farmer, A. (1977) 'Stop Cognate Production Patterns in Adult Athetotic Cerebral Palsied Speakers', *Folia Phoniatrica, 29,* 154-62.

Farmer, A. (1980) 'Voice Onset Time in Cerebral Palsied Speakers', *Folia Phoniatrica, 32,* 267-73.

Farmer, A. and Brayton, E.R. (1979) 'Speech Characteristics of Fluent and Dysfluent Down's Syndrome Adults', *Folia Phoniatrica, 31,* 284-90.

Farmer, A. and Florance, K.M. (1977) 'Segmental Duration Differences: Language Disordered and Normal Children' in Andrews, J. and Burns, M.S. (eds.), *Selected Papers in Language Disorders,* vol. 2, Institute for Continuing Professional Education, Evanston, Ill.

Farmer, A. and Green, W.B. (1978) 'Differential Effects of Auditory Masking on Cerebral Palsied Speakers', *Journal of Phonetics, 6,* 127-32.

Farmer, A. and Lencione, R.M. (1977) 'A Prevocalization in Cerebral Palsied Speakers: Durational and Articulatory Analyses', *British Journal of Disorders of Communication, 12,* 109-18.

Farmer, A., Lencione, R.M., Rothenberg, M. and O'Connell, E.J. Jr. (1976) 'Diagnostic Value of a Prevocalization in the Speech of Athetotic Cerebral Palsied Speakers', *Proceedings XVI — The International Congress on Logopedics and Phoniatrics,* S. Karger, Basel.

Feinberg, L.R. (1981) 'Perception of Temporally Distorted Sentential Approximations of varying length by Normal Learning Children and Children with Auditory Processing Deficits', unpublished M.A. thesis, Memphis State University, Memphis, Tennessee.

Feinstein, B. (1945/6) 'The Application of Electromyography to Affections of the Facial and the Intrinsic Laryngeal Muscles', *Proceedings of the Royal Society of Medicine, 39,* 817.

Fenn, W.O. (1958) Quoted in Campbell, E.J.M. (1958) *The Respiratory Muscles,* Lloyd-Luke, London.

Finley, W.W., Niman, C., Standley, J. and Ender, P. (1976) 'Frontal EMG-biofeedback Training of Athetoid Cerebral Palsy Patients', *Biofeedback and Self-Regulations, 1,* 169-82.

Finley, W.W., Niman, C., Standley, J. and Wansley, R.A. (1977) 'Electrophysiologic Behaviour Modification of Frontal EMG in Cerebral-palsied Children', *Biofeedback and Self-Regulations, 2,* 59-79.

Fisher, L. (1980) 'Learning Disabilities and Auditory Processing' in Van Hattum, R. (ed.), *The Speech Language Pathologist in the Schools,* C.C. Thomas, Springfield, Illinois.

Fleisch, A. (1925) *Pneumotachograph: Apparatus for Recording Respiratory Flow,* Archiv für die gesamte Physiologie, 209: 713.

Fletcher, H. (1965) *Speech and Hearing in Communication*, Van Nostrand, New York.

Fónagy, I. (1976) 'La Mimique Buccale. Aspect Radiologique de la Vive Voix', *Phonetica*, *33*, 31-44.

Forster, F. (1962) *Synopsis of Neurology*, Mosby, St. Louis, MO.

Foulke, E. (1966) 'Comparison of Comprehension of Two Forms of Compressed Speech', *Journal of Exceptional Children*, *33*, 169-73.

Foulke, E. (1971) 'The Perception of Time-compressed Speech' in Horton, D. and Jenkins, J. (eds.), *The Perception of Language*, Charles E. Merrill, Columbus, Ohio.

Fourcin, A.J. (1974) 'Laryngographic Examination of Vocal Fold Vibration' in Wyke, B. (ed.), *Ventilatory and Phonatory Control Systems*, Oxford University Press, London.

Fourcin, A.J. (1978) 'Acoustic Patterns and Speech Acquisition' in Waterson, N. and Snow, C. (eds.), *The Development of Communication*, J. Wiley, London.

Fourcin, A.J. (1980) 'Speech Pattern Audiometry' in Beagley, H.A. (ed.), *Auditory Investigation: the Scientific and Technological Basis*, Clarendon Press, Oxford.

Fourcin, A.J. (1982) 'Laryngographic Assessment of Phonatory Function' in Ludlow, C.K. (ed.), *Proceedings of the Conference on the Assessment of Vocal Pathology, ASHA Reports, 11,* Maryland, 116-27.

Fourcin, A.J. and Abberton, E. (1971) 'First Applications of a New Laryngograph', *Medical and Biological Review*, *21*, 172-82.

Fourcin, A.J. and Abberton, E. (1972) 'First Applications of a New Laryngograph', *Volta Review*, *74*, 161-76.

Fourcin, A.J. and Abberton, E. (1976) 'The Laryngograph and Voiscope in Speech Therapy' in Loebell, E. (ed.), *Proceedings of the XVI International Congress of Logopaedics and Phoniatrics*, S. Karger, Basel, 116-22.

Fourcin, A.J. and Abberton, E. (1980) 'First Applications of a New Laryngograph' in Pickett, H., Levitt, J.M. and Houde, R.A. (eds.), *Sensory Aids for the Hearing Impaired*, J. Wiley, New York.

Fourcin, A.J., Douek, E.E., Moore, B.C.J., Rosen, S.M., Walliker, J.R., Howard, D.M., Abberton, E. and Frampton, S. (1983) 'Speech Perception with Promontory Stimulation', *Annals of the New York Academy of Sciences, 4,* 280-94.

Fourcin, A.J., Rosen, S.M., Moore, B.C.J., Clarke, G.P., Dodson, H. and Bannister, L.H. (1978) 'External Electrical Stimulation of the Cochlea: Clinical, Psychophysical, Speech Perceptual and Histological Findings', *British Journal of Audiology*, *13*, 85-107.

Frank, J.S., Williams, I.D. and Hayes, K.C. (1977) 'The Ischemic Nerve Block and Skilled Movement', *Journal of Motor Behavior*, *9*, 217-24.

Freeman, B.A. (1977) 'Studies Using Time-compressed/Expanded Monosyllables and Sentential Approximations as Measures of Central Auditory Pathology', seminar presented to the New York Speech and Hearing Association Meeting, Rochester, New York.

Freeman, B.A. and Beasley, D.S. (1978) 'Discrimination of Time-altered Sentential Approximations and Monosyllables by Children with Reading Problems', *Journal of Speech and Hearing Research*, *21*, 497-506.

Freeman, B.A. and Church, G. (1977) 'Recall and Repetition of Time-compressed Sentential Approximations', *Journal of the American Audiology Society, 3,* 47-50.

Freeman, F.J., Sands, E.S. and Harris, K.S. (1978) 'Temporal Co-ordination of Phonation and Articulation in a Case of Verbal Apraxia: a Voice Onset Time Study', *Brain and Language*, *6*, 106-11.

Freeman, F.J. and Ushijima, T. (1978) 'Laryngeal Muscle Activity During Stuttering', *Journal of Speech and Hearing Research*, *21*, 538-62.

Froeschels, E. (1943) 'Hygiene of the Voice', *Archives of Otolaryngology, 38,* 122-30.

Fucci, D.J., Hall, D.E. and Weiner, F.F. (1971) 'Normative Study of Oral and Nonoral Structures Using Vibrotactile Stimuli', *Perceptual Motor Skills*, *33*, 1099-105.

Fucci, D.J. and Robertson, J.H. (1971) ' "Functional" Defective Articulation on Oral Sensory Disturbance', *Perceptual Motor Skills*, *33*, 711-4.

Fujita, K. (1966) 'Pathophysiology of the Larynx from the Viewpoint of Phonation', *Journal of the Japanese Society of Otorhinolaryngology*, *69*, 459.

Gardner, H., Albert, M. and Weintraub, S. (1975) 'Comprehending a Word: the Influence of Speed and Redundancy on Auditory Comprehension in Aphasia', *Cortex*, *11*, 155-62.

Garvey, W.D. (1953) 'The Intelligibility of Speeded Speech', *Journal of Experimental Psychology, 45,* 102-8.

Gay, T., Hirose, H., Strome, M. and Sawashima, M. (1972) 'Electromyography of the Intrinsic Laryngeal Muscles During Phonation', *Annals of Otology, Rhinology and Laryngology*, *81*, 401-9.

Geffen, G. (1976) 'Development of Hemispheric Specialization for

Speech Perception', *Cortex, 12*, 337-46.

Gerver, D. (1969) 'Effects of Grammaticalness, Presentation Rate, and Message Length on Auditory Short-term Memory', *Quarterly Journal of Experimental Psychology, 21*, 203-8.

Geschwind, N. (1965) 'Disconnection Syndromes in Animals and in Man, Part II', *Brain, 88*, 585-644.

Gibson, J.J. (1962) 'Observations on Active Touch', *Psychological Review, 69*, 477-90.

Gilbert, H.R. and Campbell, M.I. (1978) 'Voice Onset Time in the Speech of Hearing-impaired Individuals', *Folia Phoniatrica, 30*, 67-81.

Glaser, E.R., Skolnick, M.L., McWilliams, B.J. and Shprintzen, R.J. (1979) 'The dynamics of Passavant's Ridge in Subjects with and without Velopharyngeal Insufficiency — a Multiview Videofluoroscopic Study', *Cleft Palate Journal, 16*, 24-33.

Goldiamond, I. (1965) 'Stuttering and Fluency as Manipulatable Operant Response Classes' in Krasner, L. and Ullman, L. (eds.), *Research in Behavior Modification*, Holt, New York.

Goodglass, H. and Peck, E.A. (1972) 'Dichotic Ear Order Effects in Korsakoff and Normal Subjects', *Neuropsychologia, 10*, 211-17.

Goodwin, G.M., McCloskey, D.I. and Matthews, P.B.C. (1972a) 'The Contribution of Muscle Afferents to Kinesthesia Shown by Vibration Induced Illustrations of Movement and by the Effects of Paralyzing Joint Afferents', *Brain, 95*, 705-48.

Goodwin, G.M., McCloskey, D.I. and Matthews, P.B.C. (1972b) 'Proprioceptive Illusions Induced by Muscle Vibration: Contribution by Muscle Spindles to Perception', *Science, 175*, 1382-84.

Gordon, M.C. (1970) 'Some Effects of Stimulus Presentation Rate and Complexity on Perception and Retention in Brain Damaged Patients', *Cortex, 6*, 723-86.

Gordon, M.T., Morton, F.M. and Simpson, J.C. (1978) 'Airflow Measurement in Diagnosis Assessment and Treatment of Mechanical Dysphonia', *Folia Phoniatrica, 30*, 161-74.

Grabb, W.C., Rosenstein, S.W. and Bzoch, K.R. (eds.) (1971) *Cleft Lip and Palate*, Little, Brown and Co., Boston.

Greene, M.C.L. (1980) *The Voice and its Disorders* (3rd edn), Pitman Medical, London.

Gregory, A.H. (1982) 'Ear Dominance for Pitch', *Neuropsychologia, 20*, 89-90.

Grossman, R.C. (1967) 'Methods of Determining Oral Tactile Experience' in Bosma, J.F. (ed.), *Symposium on Oral Sensation and*

Perception, Charles C. Thomas, Springfield, Ill.

Grossman, R.C. and Hattis, B.F. (1967) 'Oral Mucosal Sensory Innervation and Sensory Experience: a Review' in Bosma, J.F. (ed.), *Symposium on Oral Sensation and Perception*, Charles C. Thomas, Springfield, Ill.

Gruber, L. and Powell, R.L. (1974) 'Responses of Stuttering and Non-stuttering Children to a Dichotic Listening Task', *Perceptual and Motor Skills*, *38*, 263-4.

Guilford, A.M. and Hawk, A.M. (1968) 'A Comparative Study of Form Identification in Neurologically Impaired and Normal Adult Subjects', *Speech and Hearing Science Research Reports,* University of Michigan.

Guitar, B. (1975) 'Reduction of Stuttering Frequency Using Analog Electromyographic Feedback', *Journal of Speech and Hearing Research*, *18*, 672-85.

Haggard, M.P. (1971) 'Encoding and the REA for Speech Signals', *Quarterly Journal of Experimental Psychology*, *23*, 34-45.

Haggard, M.P. and Parkinson, A.M. (1971) 'Stimulus and Task Factors as Determinants of Ear Advantages', *Quarterly Journal of Experimental Psychology*, *23*, 168-77.

Haines, R.W. (1932) 'The Laws of Muscle and Tendon Growth', *Journal of Anatomy*, *66*, 578-85.

Haines, R.W. (1934) 'On Muscles of Full and Short Action', *Journal of Anatomy*, *69*, 20-4.

Haldane, J.S. and Priestly, J.G. (1905) 'The Regulation of Lung Volume', *Journal of Physiology*, *32*, 255-66.

Hall, J.L. and Goldstein, M.H. (1968) 'Representation of Binaural Stimuli by Single Units in Primary Auditory Cortex of Unanesthetized Cats', *Journal of the Acoustical Society of America*, *43*, 456-61.

Hambly, R.M. and Farmer, A. (1982) 'An Analysis of Vowel Duration in a Group of Language Disordered Children Exhibiting the Open Syllable Pattern', *Folia Phoniatrica, 34,* 65-70.

Hand, C.R., Barns, M.O. and Ireland, E. (1979) 'Treatment of Hypertonicity in Muscles of Lip Retraction', *Biofeedback and Self-Regulations*, *4*, 171-81.

Hanna, R., Wilfling, F. and McNeil, B. (1975) 'A Biofeedback Treatment for Stuttering', *Journal of Speech and Hearing Disorders*, *40*, 270-3.

Hardcastle, J. (1976) *Physiology of Speech Production*, Academic Press, London.

Hardy, J.C. (1970) 'Development of Neuromuscular Systems Underlying Speech Production' in Wertz, R.T. (ed.), *Speech and the
Dentofacial Complex: The State of the Art,* American Speech
and Hearing Association, Washington, DC.

Hardy, J.C., Netsell, R., Schweiger, J.W. and Morris, H.L. (1969)
'Management of Velopharyngeal Dysfunction in Cerebral Palsy',
Journal of Speech and Hearing Disorders, 34, 123-37.

Harris, J., Haines, H., Kelsey, P. and Clark, T. (1961) 'The Relation
Between Speech Intelligibility and the Electro-acoustic Characteristics of Low-fidelity Circuitry', *Journal of Auditory Research,
1,* 357-81.

Harris, K.S. (1981) 'Electromyography as a Technique for Laryngeal
Investigation' in *Proceedings of the Conference on the Assessment
of Vocal Pathology, ASHA Reports, 11,* 70-87.

Hartley, X.Y. (1981) 'Lateralisation of Speech Stimuli in Young
Down's Syndrome Children', *Cortex, 17,* 241-8.

Haskins, J. (1949) 'A Phonetically-balanced Test of Speech Discrimination for Children', unpublished M.A. thesis, Northwestern University.

Hayden, M.E., Kirsten, E. and Singh, S. (1979) 'Role of Distinctive
Features in Dichotic Presentation of 21 English Consonants', *Journal
of the Acoustical Society of America, 65,* 1039-46.

Hellyer, N.L. and Farmer, A. (1982) 'A Comparison of Vowel Formant Measurements Between Post-tracheoctomy and Post-babbling
Children', *Folia Phoniatrica, 34,* 115-19.

Henke, W. (1967) 'Preliminaries to Speech Synthesis Based Upon an
Articulary Model', paper presented at the Conference on Speech
Communications and Processing, Cambridge, Mass.

Hewlett, N. and Anthony, J. (1982) 'Airflow and Voicing Characteristics in Some Segment Types', *Work in Progress, 15, Department
of Linguistics, University of Edinburgh,* 102-8.

Hillman, R. and Gilbert, H. (1977) 'Voice Onset Time for Voiceless
Stop Consonants in the Fluent Reading of Stutterers and Non-
stutterers', *Journal of the Acoustical Society of America, 61,* 610-1.

Hirano, M., Koike, Y. and Joyner, J. (1969) 'Style of Phonation: an
Electromyographic Investigation of Some Laryngeal Muscles',
Archives of Otolaryngology, 89, 902-7.

Hirano, M., Vennard, W. and Ohala, J. (1970) 'Regulation of Register,
Pitch, and Intensity of Voice', *Folia Phoniatrica, 22,* 1-20.

Hirose, H., Kiritani, S., Ushijima, T. and Sawashima, M. (1978) 'Analysis of Abnormal Articulatory Dynamics in Two Dysarthric Patients',
Journal of Speech and Hearing Disorders, 43, 96-105.

Hirose, H., Kiritani, S., Ushijima, T., Yoshioka, H. and Sawashima, M. (1981) 'Patterns of Dysarthric Movements in Patients with Parkinsonism', *Folia Phoniatrica*, *33*, 204-15.

Hiroto, I. (1980) 'An x-ray Study on the Level of the Vocal Fold during Phonation', paper presented at XVIII Congress of the International Association of Logopedics and Phoniatrics, Washington, DC.

Hirsh, I. (1967) 'Information Processing in Input Channels for Speech and Language: the Significance of Serial Order of Stimuli' in Millikan, C. and Darley, F. (eds.), *Brain Mechanism Underlying Speech and Language*, Grune and Stratton, New York.

Hirsh, I., Davis, H., Silverman, S., Reynolds, E., Eldert, E. and Benson, R. (1952) 'Development of Materials for Speech Audiometry', *Journal of Speech and Hearing Disorders*, *17*, 321-37.

Hochberg, I. and Kabcenell, J. (1967) 'Oral Stereognosis in Normal and Cleft Palate Individuals', *Cleft Palate Journal*, *4*, 47-57.

Hollien, H. (1974) 'On Vocal Registers', *Journal of Phonetics*, *2*, 125-44.

Houk, J.C. and Henneman, E. (1967) 'Responses of Golgi Tendon Organs to Active Contractions of the Soleus Muscle of the Cat', *Journal of Neurophysiology*, *30*, 466-81.

House, A.S. and Fairbanks, G. (1953) 'The Influence of Consonant Environment upon the Secondary Acoustical Characteristics of Vowels', *Journal of the Acoustical Society of America*, *25*, 105-13.

Huffman, A.L. (1978) 'Biofeedback Treatment of Orofacial Dysfunction: a Preliminary Study', *The American Journal of Occupational Therapy*, *32*, 149-54.

Huggins, A.W.F. (1967) 'Accurate Delays for Auditory Feedback Experiments', *Quarterly Journal of Experimental Psychology*, *19*, 78-80.

Husson, N. (1950) 'Etudes des Phénomèmes Physiologiques et Acoustiques Foundamentaux de la voix Chantée', unpublished thesis, Paris.

Iglesias, A., Kuehn, D.P. and Morris, H.L. (1980) 'Simultaneous Assessment of Pharyngeal Wall and Velar Displacement for Selected Speech Sounds', *Journal of Speech and Hearing Research*, *23*, 429-46.

Inglis, J., Campbell, D. and Donald, M. (1977) 'Electromyographic Biofeedback and Neuromuscular Rehabilitation' in Kamiya, J. *et al.* (eds.), *Biofeedback and Self-Control*, Aldine, Chicago.

Inman, V.T., Saunders, J.B. and Abbott, L.C. (1944) 'Observations on the Functions of the Shoulder Joint', *Journal of Bone and Joint Surgery*, *26*, 1-30.

Isshiki, N. and von Leden, H. (1964) 'Hoarseness: Aerodynamic Studies', *Archives of Otolaryngology*, *80*, 206-13.

Itoh, M., Sasanuma, S., Hirose, H., Yoshioka, H. and Ushijima, T. (1980) 'Abnormal Articulatory Dynamics in a Patient with Apraxia of Speech: x-ray Microbeam Observation', *Brain and Language*, *11*, 66-75.

Itoh, M., Sasanuma, S. and Ushijima, T. (1979) 'Velar Movements During Speech in a Patient with Apraxia of Speech', *Brain and Language*, *7*, 227-39.

Iwota, S. and von Leden, H. (1970) 'Voiceprints in Laryngeal Disease', *Archives of Otolaryngology*, *91*, 74-80.

Jerger, J. (1964) 'Auditory Tests for Disorders of the Central Auditory Mechanism' in Field, W. and Alford, B. (eds.), *Neurological Aspects of Auditory and Vestibular Disorders*, Thomas, Springfield.

Jerger, J. (1970) 'Diagnostic Significance of SSI Test Procedures: Retrocochlear Site' in Rojskger, C. (ed.), *Speech Audiometry (Second Danavox Symposium)*, Danavox Foundation, Odense, Denmark.

Johns, D.F. and La Pointe, L.L. (1976) 'Neurogenic Disorders of Output Processing: Apraxia of Speech' in Whitaker, H. and Whitaker, H.A. (eds.), *Studies in Neurolinguistics*, vol. 1, Academic Press, New York.

Johnson, J.P., Sommers, R.K. and Weidner, W.E. (1977) 'Dichotic Ear Preference in Aphasia', *Journal of Speech and Hearing Research*, *20*, 116-29.

Jones, D. (1950) *The Phoneme, its Nature and its Use*, Heffer, Cambridge.

Katz, J. (1962) 'The Use of Staggered Spondee Words for Assessing the Integrity of the Central Auditory Nervous System', *Journal of Auditory Research*, *2*, 327-37.

Kawamura, Y. (1970) 'A Role of Oral Afferents for Mandibular and Lingual Movements' in Bosma, J.F. (ed.), *Second Symposium on Oral Sensation and Perception*, Charles C. Thomas, Springfield, Ill.

Keller, K.C. (1971) *Instrumental Articulatory Phonetics: An Introduction to Techniques and Results*, Summer Institute of Linguistics, University of Oklahoma.

Kelman, A.W., Gordon, M.T., Morton, F.M. and Simpson, I.C. (1981) 'Comparison of Methods for Assessing Vocal Function', *Folia Phoniatrica*, *33*, 51-65.

Kelman, A.W., Gordon, M.T., Simpson, I.C. and Morton, F.M. (1975) 'Assessment of Vocal Function by Airflow Measurements', *Folia Phoniatrica*, *27*, 250-62.

Kelso, J.A.S. (1977) 'Motor Control Mechanisms Underlying Human Movement Production', *Journal of Experimental Psychology: Human Perception and Performance*, *3*, 529-43.

Kent, R. and Netsell, R. (1975) 'A Case Study of an Ataxic Dysarthric: Cineradiographic and Spectrographic Observations', *Journal of Speech and Hearing Disorders*, *40*, 115-34.

Kent, R., Netsell, R. and Abbs, J.H. (1979) 'Acoustic Characteristics of Dysarthria Associated with Cerebellar Disease', *Journal of Speech and Hearing Research*, *22*, 627-48.

Kent, R. and Rosenbek, J.C. (1982) 'Prosodic Disturbance and Neurologic Lesion', *Brain and Language*, *15*, 259-91.

Keslinger, F. (1973) *Foundations of Behavioural Research*, Holt, Rinehart and Winston, New York.

Kimura, D. (1961) 'Cerebral Dominance and the Perception of Verbal Stimuli', *Canadian Journal of Psychology*, *15*, 166-71.

Kimura, D. (1963) 'Speech Lateralization in Young Children as Determined by an Auditory List', *Journal of Comparative and Physiological Psychology*, *56*, 599-602.

Kimura, D. (1964) 'Left-right Differences in the Perception of Melodies', *Quarterly Journal of Experimental Psychology*, *16*, 355-8.

Kimura, D. (1967) 'Functional Asymmetry of the Brain in Dichotic Listening', *Cortex*, *3*, 163-78.

King, A. and Parker, A. (1980) 'The Relevance of Prosodic Features to Speech Work with Hearing Impaired Children' in Jones, F.M. (ed.), *Language Disability in Children*, M.T.P. Press, Lancaster.

King, K.M. and Weston, P.L. (1974) 'The Effect of the Percentage of Time-compression, Sentence Length, and Age on Children's Recall Performance of Well-formed Sentences', paper presented at the American Speech and Hearing Association Convention, Las Vegas, Nevada.

Kinsbourne, M. (1975) 'The Ontogeny of Cerebral Dominance' in Aaronson, O. and Reiber, R.W. (eds.), *Developmental Psycholinguistics and Communication Disorders*, vol. 263, New York Academy of Sciences, New York.

Kiritani, S., Itoh, K. and Fujimura, O. (1975) 'Tongue-pellet Tracking by a Computer-controlled x-ray Microbeam System', *Journal of the Acoustical Society of America*, *57*, 1516-20.

Klumpp, R.G. and Webster, J.C. (1961) 'Intelligibility of Time-compressed Speech', *Journal of the Acoustical Society of America*, *33*, 265-7.

Knox, C. and Kimura, D. (1970) 'Cerebral Processing of Nonverbal Sounds in Boys and Girls', *Neuropsychologia*, *8*, 227-37.

Konkle, D.F., Beasley, D.S. and Bess, F. (1977a) 'Intelligibility of Time-altered Speech in Relation to Chronological Aging', *Journal of Speech and Hearing Research*, *20*, 108-15.

Konkle, D.F., Freeman, B.A., Riggs, D., Riensche, L.L. and Beasley, D.S. (1977b) 'Calibration Procedures for Time-compressed/expanded Speech' in Foulke, E. (ed.), *Proceedings of the Third Louisville Conference on Time-Compressed Speech*, University of Louisville, Louisville.

Kuehn, D.P. and Tomblin, J.B. (1977) 'A Cineradiographic Investigation of Children's w/r Substitutions', *Journal of Speech and Hearing Disorders*, *42*, 462-73.

Kuehn, D.P. and Van Demark, D.R. (1978) 'Assessment of Velopharyngeal Competency Following Teflon Pharyngoplasty', *Cleft Palate Journal*, *15*, 145-9.

Kuhl, P. and Speaks, C. (1972) 'Temporal Processing of Speech', paper presented at the meeting of the Acoustical Society of America, Buffalo, NY.

Künzel, H.J. (1979) 'Röntgenvideographische Evaluierung eines photoelektrischen Verfahrens zur Registrierung der Velumhöhe beim Sprechen', *Folia Phoniatrica*, *31*, 153-66.

Kurdziel, S., Noffsinger, D. and Olsen, W. (1976) 'Performance by Cortical Lesion Patients on 40 and 60% Time-compressed Materials', *Journal of the American Audiology Society*, *2*, 3-7.

Kurdziel, S., Rintelmann, W.F. and Beasley, D.S. (1975) 'Performance of Noice-induced Hearing-impaired Listeners on Time-compressed CNC Monosyllables', *Journal of the American Audiology Society*, *1*, 54-60.

Ladefoged, P. and McKinney, N.P. (1963) 'Loudness, Sound Pressure, and Sub-glottal Pressure in Speech', *Journal of the Acoustical Society of America*, *35*, 454-60.

Landman, G.H.M. (1970) *Laryngography and Cinelaryngography*, Excerpta Medica Foundation, Amsterdam.

Landt, H., and Fransson, B. (1975) 'Oral Ability to Recognize Forms and Oral Muscular Coordination Ability in Dentulous Young and Elderly Adults', *Journal of Oral Rehabilitation*, *2*, 125-38.

Lanyon, R.J., Barrington, C.C. and Newman, A.C. (1976) 'Modification of Stuttering Through EMG Biofeedback: a Preliminary

Study', *Behavior Therapy*, 7, 96-103.

LaPointe, L.L., Williams, W. and Faircloth, B.H. (1976) 'Intraoral Shape Recognition by 138 Mentally Retarded Subjects', *Perceptual Motor Skills*, 42, 19-26.

Lasky, E.Z., Weidner, W.E. and Johnson, J.P. (1976) 'Influence of Linguistic Complexity, Rate of Presentation, and Interphase Pause Time on Auditory-verbal Comprehension of Adult Aphasic Patients', *Brain and Language*, 3, 386-95.

Lass, N.J. (ed.) (1974) *Experimental Phonetics*, M.S.S. Information Corporation, Arno Press, New York.

Lass, N.J., Bell, R.R., Simcoe, J.C., McClung, N.J. and Park, W.E. (1972) 'Assessment of Oral Tactile Perception: Some Methodological Considerations', *Central States Speech Journal*, 23, 165-73.

Lass, N.J. and Clay, T.H. (1973) 'The Effect of Memory on Subject Performance on a Test of Oral Form Discrimination', *Western Speech*, 37, 27-33.

Lass, N.J. and Foulke, E. (1976) 'The Use of Time-expanded Speech as an Aid in the Diagnosis of Articulation Disorders', *Journal of Communication Disorders, 9,* 111-19.

Lass, N.J., Kotchek, C.L. and Deem, J.F. (1972) 'Oral Two Point Discrimination: Further Evidence of Asymmetry on Right and Left Sides of Selected Oral Structures', *Perceptual Motor Skills*, 35, 59-67.

Lass, N.J. and Park, W.E. (1973) 'Oral Two Point Discrimination: Consistency of Two-point Limens on Selected Oral Sites', *Perceptual Motor Skills*, 37, 881-2.

Lass, N.J., Tekieli, M.E. and Eye, M.P. (1971) 'A Comparative Study of Two Procedures for Assessment of Oral Tactile Perception', *Central States Speech Journal*, 22, 21-6.

Laughlin, S.A., Naeser, M.A. and Gordon, W.P. (1979) 'Effects of Three Syllable Durations using the Melodic Intonation Therapy Technique', *Journal of Speech and Hearing Research*, 22, 311-20.

Leanderson, R., Persson, A. and Ohman, S. (1970) 'Electromyographic Studies of the Facial Muscles in Dysarthria', *Acta Oto-Laryngologica*, 263, 89-94.

Lee, B.S. (1950a) 'Some Effects of Sidetone Delay', *Journal of the Acoustical Society of America*, 22, 639-40.

Lee, B.S. (1950b) 'Effects of Delayed Speech Feedback', *Journal of the Acoustical Society of America*, 22, 824-6.

Lee, F.F. (1972) 'Time Compression and Expansion of Speech by the

Sampling Method', *Journal of Audio Engineering Society, 20*, 738-42.

Leeper, H.A., Nieurvesteeg, Y., Bishop, L., Lass, N.J. and Beekwith, S. (1980) 'The Use of Time-expanded Speech in Judgements of Hypernasality', *Journal of Communication Disorders, 13*, 335-9.

Leff, J. and Abberton, E. (1981) 'Voice Pitch Measurements in Schizophrenia and Depression', *Psychological Medicine, 11*, 849-52.

Lehiste, I. (1965) 'Some Acoustic Characteristics of Dysarthric Speech', *Bibliotheca Phonetica 2*, Karger, Basel.

Lehiste, I. (ed.) (1967) *Readings in Acoustic Phonetics*, MIT Press, Cambridge, MA.

Lehiste, I. (1976) 'Suprasegmental Features of Speech' in Lass, N.J. (ed.), *Contemporary Issues in Experimental Phonetics*, Academic Press, New York.

Lenneberg, E.H. (1967) *Biological Foundations of Language*, Wiley, New York.

Levine, S.I. (1965) 'A Study of Performance of Normal Subjects and Aphasic Subjects in Tests of Oral and Manual Stereognosis', unpublished Master's thesis, Ohio State University.

Lewis, M.B. and Pahayan, H.M. (1980) 'The Effects of Pharyngeal Flap Surgery on Lateral Wall Motion: a Videoradiographic Evaluation', *Cleft Palate Journal, 17*, 301-4.

Liberman, A.M. (1957) 'Some Results of Research on Speech Perception', *Journal of the Acoustical Society of America, 29*, 117-23.

Liberman, A.M., Cooper, F.S., Shankweiler, D. and Studdert-Kennedy, M. (1967) 'Perception of the Speech Code', *Psychological Review, 74*, 431-61.

Lieberman, P. (1977) *Speech Physiology and Acoustic Phonetics*, MacMillan, New York.

Liles, B.Z. and Brookshire, R.H. (1975) 'The Effects of Pause Time on Auditory Comprehension of Aphasic Subjects', *Journal of Communication Disorders, 8*, 221-35.

Linebaugh, C.W. (1978) 'Dichotic Ear Preference in Aphasia: Another View', *Journal of Speech and Hearing Research, 21*, 598-600.

Lippold, O.C.J. (1967) 'Electromyography' in Verrables, P.H. and Martin, I. (eds.), *A Manual of Psychophysiological Methods*, John Wiley, New York.

Lisker, L. and Abramson, A.D. (1964) 'A Cross-language Study of Voicing in Initial Stops: Acoustic Measurements', *Word, 20*, 384-422.

Locke, J.L. (1968) 'Oral Perception and Articulation Learning', *Per-

ceptual Motor Skills, *26*, 1259-64.

Lotzmann, G. (1961) 'On the Use of Varied Delay Times in Stammering', *Folia Phoniatrica*, *13*, 276-310.

Low, J.M. and Lindsay, D.D. (1979) 'A Body-worn Delayed Auditory Feedback Fluency Aid for Stammerers', *Journal of Biomedical Engineering*, *1*, 235-9.

Lozano, R.A. and Dreyer, D.E. (1978) 'Some Effects of Delayed Auditory Feedback on Dyspraxia of Speech', *Journal of Communication Disorders*, *11*, 407-15.

Lubker, J.F. (1970) 'Aerodynamic and Ultrasonic Assessment Techniques in Speech-dentofacial Research', *ASHA Report*, *5* (Workshop on Speech and the Dentofacial Complex: State of the Art).

Lubker, J.F. and Moll, K.L. (1965) 'Simultaneous Oral-nasal Airflow Measurements and Cinefluorographic Observations During Speech Production', *Cleft Palate Journal*, *2*, 257-72.

Lubker, J.F. and Schweiger, J.W. (1969) 'Nasal Airflow as an Index of Success of Prosthetic Management of Cleft Palate', *Journal of Dental Research*, *48*, 368-75.

Luchsinger, R. and Arnold, G.E. (1965) *Voice – Speech – Language*, Constable and Co., London.

Luria, A.R. and Hutton, T. (1977) 'Modern Assessment of the Basic Forms of Aphasia', *Brain and Language*, *4*, 129-51.

Luterman, D.M., Welsh, O.L. and Melrose, J. (1966) 'Responses of Aged Males to Time-altered Speech Stimuli', *Journal of Speech and Hearing Research*, *9*, 226-30.

Lyndes, K.O. (1975) 'The Application of Biofeedback to Functional Dysphonia', *The Journal of Bio-feedback*, *2*, 12-15.

McCall, G.N. (1965, 1966) 'An Approach to the Assessment of Oral Sensation and Perception', unpublished article based on papers presented to the Louisiana Speech and Hearing Association.

McCall, G.N. and Cunningham, N.M. (1971) 'Two Point Discrimination: Asymmetry in Spatial Discrimination on Two Sides of the Tongue, a Preliminary Report', *Perceptual Motor Skills*, *32*, 368-70.

McCall, G.N. and Morgan, N.R. (1967) 'Two Point Discrimination: Two Point Limens on the Tip and Lateral Margins of the Tongue', unpublished paper presented at American Speech and Hearing Association Convention in Chicago.

McCroskey, R.L. Jr. (1958) 'The Relative Contribution of Auditory and Tactile Cues to Certain Aspects of Speech', *Southern Speech Journal*, *24*, 84-90.

McCroskey, R.L., Corley, N.W.. and Jackson, G. (1959) 'Some Effects of Disruptive Tactile Cues Upon the Production of Consonants', *Southern Speech Journal*, *25*, 55-60.

MacCurtain, F. (1981) 'Pharyngeal Factors Influencing Voice Quality', unpublished PhD thesis, University of London.

McDonald, E.T. (1964) *Articulation Testing and Treatment: A Sensory-Motor Approach*, Stanwix House Inc., Pittsburgh, PA.

McDonald, E.T. and Aungst, L.F. (1967) 'Studies in Oral Sensorimotor Function' in Bosma, J.F. (ed.), *Symposium on Oral Sensation and Perception*, Charles C. Thomas, Springfield, Ill.

McDonald, E.T. and Aungst, L.F. (1970) 'An Abbreviated Test of Oral Stereognosis' in Bosma, J.F. (ed.), *Second Symposium on Oral Sensation and Perception*, Charles C. Thomas, Springfield, Ill.

Mackay, D. (1968) 'Metamorphosis of a Critical Interval: Age-linked Changes in the Delay of Auditory Feedback that Produces Maximum Disruption of Speech', *Journal of the Acoustical Society of America*, *43*, 811-21.

McLain, J.R. (1962) 'A Comparison of Two Methods of Producing Rapid Speech', *International Journal for the Education of the Blind*, *12*, 40-3.

MacMillan, A.S. and Kelemen, G. (1952) 'Radiography of the Supraglottal Speech Organs. A Survey', *A.M.A. Archives of Otolaryngology*, *55*, 671-88.

MacNeilage, P.F. (1970) 'Motor Control of Serial Ordering of Speech', *Psychological Review*, *77*, 182-96.

McNutt, J.C. (1977) 'Oral Sensory and Motor Behaviors of Children with /s/ and /r/ Misarticulation', *Journal of Speech and Hearing Research*, *20*, 694-703.

Madison, C.I. and Fucci, D.J. (1971) 'Speech Discrimination and Tactile Kinesthetic Discrimination in Reference to Speech Production', *Perceptual Motor Skills*, *33*, 831-8.

Mahaffey, R.D. and Stromsta, C.P. (1965) 'The Effects of Auditory Feedback as a Function of Frequency, Intensity, Time and Sex', *De Therapia Vocis et Loquelae*, *2*, 233-5.

Maki, J.E., Beasley, D.S., Shoup, J. and Bess, F. (1976) 'Speech Discrimination and Response Latency of Normal-hearing and Hearing-impaired Children as a Function of Time Compression', paper presented at the American Speech and Hearing Association Convention, Houston, Texas.

Malmberg, B. (ed.) (1968) *Manual of Phonetics*, North Holland, Amsterdam.

Manning, W.H., Johnston, K. and Beasley, D.S. (1977) 'The Performance of Children with Auditory Perceptual Disorders on a Time-
compressed Speech Discrimination Measure', *Journal of Speech
and Hearing Disorders, 42*, 77-84.

Manning, W.H., Lee, B.A. and Lass, N.J. (1978) 'The Use of Time-
expanded Speech in the Identification of Part-word Repetitions of
Stutterers', *Journal of Communication Disorders, 11*, 11-15.

Manning, W.H. and Riensche, L.L. (1976) 'Auditory Assembly Abilities
of Stuttering and Nonstuttering Children', *Journal of Speech and
Hearing Research, 19*, 777-83.

Mason, R.M. (1967) 'Studies of Oral Perception Involving Subjects
with Alterations in Anatomy and Physiology' in Bosma, J.F. (ed.),
Symposium on Oral Sensation and Perception, Charles C. Thomas,
Springfield, Ill.

Menzies, R. (1790) *Tentamen Physiologicum Inaugurale de Respira-
tione*, Creech, Edinburgh.

Mescik, J., Smith, J., Hamm, N., Diffenbacker, K. and Brown, E.
(1972) 'Short-term Retention of Auditory Sequences as a Function of Stimulus Duration, Interstimulus Interval, and Encoding
Technique', *Journal of Experimental Psychology, 96*, 147-51.

Metz, D., Conture, E. and Caruso, A. (1979a) 'Voice Onset Time,
Frication and Aspiration During Stutterers' Fluent Speech', *Journal
of Speech and Hearing Research, 22*, 649-56.

Metz, D., Conture, E.G. and Colton, R.H. (1976) 'Temporal Relations
Between the Respiratory and Laryngeal Systems Prior to Stuttered Disfluencies', *ASHA, 18*, 664 (abstract).

Metz, D., Onufrak, J.A. and Ogburn, R.S. (1979b) 'An Acoustical
Analysis of Stutterer's Speech Prior to and at the Termination
of Speech Therapy', *Journal of Fluency Disorders, 4*, 249-54.

Miller, G.A. (1956) 'The Magical Number Seven, Plus or Minus Two:
Some Limits to our Capacity for Processing Information', *Psychological Review, 63*, 81-97.

Milner, B., Taylor, L. and Sperry, R. (1968) 'Lateralized Suppression
of Dichotically Presented Digits after Commissural Section in
Man', *Science, 161*, 184-6.

Mlcoch, A.G. and Noll, J.D. (1980) 'Speech Production Models as
Related to the Concept of Apraxia of Speech' in Lass, N.J. (ed.),
Speech and Language: Advances in Basic Research and Practice,
vol. 4, Academic Press, New York.

Moll, K.L. (1965) 'Photographic and Radiographic Procedures in
Speech Research', *ASHA Reports, 1*, 129-39.

Monsen, R.B. (1974) 'Duration Aspects of Vowel Production in the Speech of Deaf Children', *Journal of Speech and Hearing Research*, *17*, 386-98.

Moore, W.H. Jr. (1978) 'Some Effects of Progressively Lowering Electromyographic Levels with Feedback Procedures on the Frequency of Stuttered Verbal Behaviours', *Journal of Fluency Disorders*, *3*, 127-38.

Moore, W.H. Jr., Cunko, C. and Flowers, P. (1979) 'Cumulative Integrated Electromyographic Activity of Selected Speech-related Muscle Groups of Nonstutterers During Massed Oral Readings', *Journal of Fluency Disorders*, *4*, 149-61.

Moore, W.H. Jr., Flowers, P. and Cunko, C. (1981) 'Some Relationships Between Adaption and Electromyographic Activity at Laryngeal and Masseter Sites in Stutterers', *Journal of Fluency Disorders*, *6*, 81-94.

Moore, W.H. Jr. and Haynes, W.O. (1980) 'Alpha Hemispheric Asymmetry and Stuttering: Some Support for a Segmentation Dysfunction Hypothesis', *Journal of Speech and Hearing Research*, *23*, 229-47.

Moore, W.H. Jr. and Weidner, W.E. (1975) 'Dichotic Word-perception of Aphasic and Normal Subjects', *Perceptual and Motor Skills*, *40*, 379-86.

Moreau, V.K. and Lass, N.J. (1974) 'A Correlational Study of Stimulability, Oral Form Discrimination and Auditory Discrimination Skills in Children', *Journal of Communication Disorders*, *7*, 269-77.

Morley, A.J. (1935) 'An Analysis of the Associative and Predisposing Factors in the Symptomatology of Stuttering', unpublished PhD thesis, State University of Iowa.

Moser, H., LaGourgue, J.R. and Class, L. (1967) 'Studies of Oral Stereognosis in Normal Blind and Deaf Subjects' in Bosma, J.F. (ed.), *Symposium on Oral Sensation and Perception*, Charles C. Thomas, Springfield, Ill.

Mountcastle, V.B. and Darian-Smith, I. (1968) 'Neural Mechanisms in Somesthesia' in Mountcastle, V.B. (ed.), *Medical Physiology*, vol. II, (12th edn), Mosby, St Louis, MO.

Mourino, A.P. and Weinberg, B. (1975) 'A Cephalometric Study of Velar Stretch in 8 and 10-year-old Children', *Cleft Palate Journal*, *12*, 417-35.

Muellerleile, S. (1981) 'Portable Delayed Auditory Feedback Device: a Preliminary Report', *Journal of Fluency Disorders*, *6*, 361-3.

Neelly, J.N. (1961) 'A Study of the Speech Behaviour of Stutterers and Non-stutterers Under Normal and Delayed Auditory Feedback', *Journal of Speech and Hearing Disorders, Monograph Supplement 7*, 63-82.

Netsell, R. (1969) 'Evaluation of Velopharyngeal Function in Dysarthria', *Journal of Speech and Hearing Disorders, 34*, 113-22.

Netsell, R. and Cleeland, C.S. (1973) 'Modification of Lip Hypertonia in Dysarthria Using EMG Feedback', *Journal of Speech and Hearing Disorders, 38*, 131-40.

Netsell, R. and Kent, R. (1976) 'Paroxysmal Ataxic Dysarthria', *Journal of Speech and Hearing Disorders, 41*, 93-109.

Newell, D. and Rugel, R.P. (1981) 'Hemispheric Specialization in Normal and Disabled Readers', *Journal of Learning Disabilities, 14*, 296-7.

Niccum, N., Rubens, A.B. and Speaks, C. (1981) 'Effects of Stimulus Material on the Dichotic Listening Performance of Aphasic Patients', *Journal of Speech and Hearing Research, 24*, 526-34.

Niimi, S. and Simada, Z. (1980) 'Ultrasonic Investigation of Tongue Configuration during Speech', paper presented at *XVIII Congress of the International Association of Logopedics and Phoniatrics*, Washington, DC.

Nikam, S., Beasley, D.S. and Rintelmann, W.F. (1976) 'Perception of Time-compression Consonant-nucleus-consonant Monosyllables by Non-native Speakers/listeners of English', *Journal of the American Audiology Society, 2*, 45-8.

Noll, M.A. (1967) 'Cepstrum Pitch Determination', *Journal of the Acoustical Society of America, 41*, 293-309.

O'Connor, J.D. and Arnold, G.F. (1973) *Intonation of Colloquial English* (2nd edn), Longman, London.

Oelschlaeger, M.L. and Orchik, D.J. (1977) 'Time-compressed Speech Discrimination in Central Auditory Disorder: a Pediatric Case Study', *Journal of Speech and Hearing Disorders, 42*, 483-6.

Ojeman, G. (1976) 'Subcortical Language Mechanisms' in Whitaker, H. and Whitaker, H.A. (eds.), *Studies in Neurolinguistics*, vol. 2, Academic Press, New York.

Orchik, D.J., Holgate, S. and Danko, M.C. (1979) 'Time-compressed Speech Discrimination, Reading Readiness, and the Effect of Clinical Method', *Audiology, 18*, 80-7.

Orchik, D.J. and Oelschlaeger, M.L. (1977) 'Time-compressed Speech Discrimination in Children and its Relationship to Articulation', *Journal of the American Audiology Society, 3*, 37-41.

Orchik, D.J., Walker, D.C. and Larson, L. (1977) 'Time-compressed

Speech Discrimination in Adult Aphasics', *Journal of Auditory Research, 17*, 205-15.

Ormson, K. and Williams, D. (1975) 'Central Auditory Function as Assessed by Time-compressed Speech with Elementary School Children Having Articulation and Reading Problems', paper presented at the American Speech and Hearing Association Convention, Washington, DC.

Orton, S.T. (1928) 'A Physiological Theory of Reading Disability and Stuttering in Children', *New England Journal of Medicine, 199*, 1045-52.

Pahn, J. (1981) 'Röntgenologische Untersuchungsmethode der Nervus-laryngeus-superior-Parese', *Folia Phoniatrica, 33,* 15-22.

Paine, R.S. (1967) 'Manual Stereognosis' in Bosma, J.F. (ed.), *Symposium on Oral Sensation and Perception*, Charles C. Thomas, Springfield, Ill.

Painter, C. (1979) *An Introduction to Instrumental Phonetics*, University Park Press, Baltimore.

Pantalos, J., Schuckers, G.H. and Hipskind, N. (1975) 'Sentence Length Duration Relationships in an Auditory Assembly Task', *Journal of Communication Disorders, 8*, 61-74.

Parkhurst, B.G. (1970) 'The Effect of Time-altered Speech Stimuli on the Performance of Right Hemiplegic Adult Aphasics', paper presented at the American Speech and Hearing Association Convention, New York.

Passy, P. (1914) *The Sounds of the French Language*, Clarendon Press, Oxford.

Patterson, J. and Riensche, L.L. (1979) 'Recency and Primacy Effects for Time Compressed Rhymed Word Sequences', paper presented at the American Speech-Language-Hearing Association Convention, Atlanta, Georgia.

Perkell, J.S. (1969) *Physiology of Speech Production: Results and Implications of a Quantitative Cineradiographic Study*, MIT Press, Cambridge, Mass.

Peterson, G.E. and Barney, H.L. (1952) 'Control Methods Used in a Study of Vowels', *Journal of the Acoustical Society of America, 24*, 175-84.

Pettit, J.M. and Noll, J.D. (1979) 'Cerebral Dominance in Aphasia Recovery', *Brain and Language, 7*, 191-200.

Pike, K.L. (1948) *Tone Languages*, University of Michigan Publications. Linguistics, vol. 4.

Portmann, G. (1957) 'The Physiology of Phonation (the Seman Lecture for 1956)', *Journal of Laryngology and Otolaryngology*, *71*, 1-15.

Potter, R.K., Kopp, G.A. and Kopp, H.G. (1966) *Visible Speech*, Dover, New York.

Pressel, G. and Hochberg, I. (1974) 'Oral Form Discrimination of Children with Cleft Palate', *Cleft Palate Journal*, *11*, 66-71.

Prior, M.R. and Bradshaw, J.L. (1979) 'Hemisphere Functioning in Autistic Children', *Cortex*, *15*, 73-81.

Prosek, R.A., Montgomery, A.A., Walden, B.E. and Schwartz, D.M. (1978) 'EMG Biofeedback in the Treatment of Hyperfunctional Voice Disorders', *Journal of Speech and Hearing Disorders*, *43*, 282-94.

Pruszewicz, A., Obrebowski, A. and Gradzki, J. (1976) 'Postmedicamentous Voice Virilisation. X-ray Examination of the Larynx' in Loebell, E. (ed.), *Proceedings XVIth International Congress of Logopedics and Phoniatrics. Interlaken 1974*, S. Karger, Basel.

Putnam, A.H.B. and Ringel, R.L. (1976) 'A Cineradiographic Study of Articulation in Two Talkers with Temporarily Induced Oral Sensory Deprivation', *Journal of Speech and Hearing Research*, *19*, 247-66.

Quigley, L.F. (1967) 'A Comparison of Airflow and Cephalometric Techniques for Evaluation of Normal and Cleft-palate Patients, Part 1', *American Journal of Orthodontics*, *53*, 423-43.

Quigley, L.F., Shiere, F.R., Webster, R.C. and Cobb, C.M. (1964) 'Measuring Palato-pharyngeal Competence with the Nasal Anemometer', *Cleft Palate Journal*, *1*, 304-13.

Quigley, L.F., Webster, R.C., Coffey, R.J., Kellerher, R.E. and Grant, H.P. (1963) 'Velocity and Volume Measurements of Nasal and Oral Airflow in Normal and Cleft-palate Speech, Utilising a Warm-wire Flowmeter and Two-channel Recorder', *Journal of Dental Research*, *42*, 1520-7.

Ranford, H.J. (1982) ' "Larynx-NAD"?', *CST Bulletin*, *359*, 5.

Razzell, R., Anthony, J. and Watson, A.C.H. (in press) 'A U.K. Survey of Subjective Judgement of Nasality'.

Reich, A.R. and Lerman, J.W. (1978) 'Teflon Laryngoplasty: an Acoustical and Perceptual Study', *Journal of Speech and Hearing Disorders*, *43*, 496-505.

Ridgway, A. and Thumm, W. (1968) *The Physics of Medical Radiography*, Addison-Wesley, Reading, Massachusetts.

Riensche, L.L. and Beasley, D.S. (1979) 'Ear Laterality Effects for Time Compressed Rhyme Sequences', paper presented at the American

Speech-Language-Hearing Association Convention, Atlanta, Georgia.

Riensche, L.L. and Clauser, P. (1982) 'Auditory Perceptual Abilities of Formerly Misarticulating Children', paper presented at the Mid-South Conference on Communicative Disorders, Memphis, Tennessee.

Riensche, L.L., Konkle, D. and Beasley, D.S. (1976) 'Discrimination of Time-compressed CNC Monosyllables by Normal Listeners', *Journal of Auditory Research, 16,* 98-101.

Riensche, L.L. and Slate, N. (1981) 'Performance of Teenagers Presented Time Compressed Sentential Stimuli', paper presented at the American Speech-Language-Hearing Association Convention, Los Angeles, California.

Riensche, L.L., Wohlert, A. and Porch, B. (1980) 'Preferred Speech Rate Relative to Comprehension Rate in Aphasia', paper presented at the American Speech-Language-Hearing Association Convention, Detroit, Michigan.

Ringel, R.L. (1970) 'Oral Sensation and Perception: a Selective Review' in Wertz, R.T. (series ed.), and Fricke, J.E. (project director), *Speech and Dentofacial Complex: The State of the Art, ASHA Report No. 5,* American Speech and Hearing Association, Washington, DC.

Ringel, R.L., Burk, K.W. and Scott, C.M. (1970a) 'Tactile Perception: Form Discrimination in the Mouth' in Bosma, J.F. (ed.), *Second Symposium on Oral Sensation and Perception,* Charles C. Thomas, Springfield, Ill.

Ringel, R.L. and Ewanowski, S.J. (1965) 'Oral Perception: I. Two Point Discrimination', *Journal of Speech and Hearing Research, 8,* 389-98.

Ringel, R.L. and Fletcher, H.M. (1967) 'Oral Perception: III. Texture Discrimination', *Journal of Speech and Hearing Research, 10,* 642-9.

Ringel, R.L., House, A.S., Burk, K.W., Dolinsky, J.P. and Scott, C.M. (1970b) 'Some Relations Between Orosensory Aspects of Speech Sound Production', *Journal of Speech and Hearing Disorders, 35,* 3-11.

Ringel, R.L., Saxman, J.H. and Brooks, A.R. (1967) 'Oral Perception: II. Mandibular Kinesthesia', *Journal of Speech and Hearing Research, 10,* 637-41.

Ringel, R.L. and Steer, M.D. (1963) 'Some Effects of Tactile Auditory Alterations on Speech Output', *Journal of Speech and Hearing Research, 6,* 369-78.

Rintelmann, W.F. and Jetty, B. (1968) Unpublished manuscript, Department of Audiology and Speech Sciences, Michigan State

University, East Lansing, Michigan.

Rontal, E., Rontal, M. and Rolnick, M.I. (1975a) 'Objective Evaluation of Vocal Pathology using Voice Spectrography', *Annals of Otolaryngology, Rhinology and Laryngology, 84*, 662-7.

Rontal, E., Rontal, M. and Rolnick, M.I. (1975b) 'The Use of Spectrograms in the Evaluation of Vocal Cord Injection', *The Laryngoscope, 85*, 47-56.

Rose, J.E. and Mountcastle, V.B. (1959) 'Touch and Kinesthesis' in Field, J., Magoun, H.W. and Hall, V.E. (eds.), *Neurophysiology*, vol. 1, American Physiological Society, Washington, DC.

Rosen, S.M., Fourcin, A.J. and Moore, B.C.J. (1981) 'Voice Pitch as an Aid to Lipreading', *Nature, 291*, 5811, 150-2.

Rosenbek, J.C., Wertz, R.T. and Darley, F.L. (1973) 'Oral Sensation and Perception in Apraxia of Speech and Aphasia', *Journal of Speech and Hearing Research, 16*, 22-36.

Rosenfield, D.B. and Goodglass, H. (1980) 'Dichotic Testing of Cerebral Dominance in Stutterers', *Brain and Language, 11*, 170-80.

Rosenweig, M.R. (1951) 'Representation of the Two Ears at the Auditory Cortex', *American Journal of Physiology, 169*, 147-58.

Ross, M. and Lerman, J. (1970) 'A Picture Identification Test for Hearing-impaired Children', *Journal of Speech and Hearing Research, 13*, 44-53.

Rothenberg, M. (1968) 'The Breath-stream Dynamics of Simple-released Plosive Production', *Bibliotheca Phonetica, 6*, Karger, Basel.

Rubin, H.J. (1960) 'Further Observations on the Neurochronaxic Theory of Voice Production', *American Medical Association Archives of Otolaryngology, 72*, 207-11.

Rubino, C.A. (1972) 'A Simple Procedure for Constructing Dichotic Listening Tapes', *Cortex, 8*, 335-8.

Ruscello, D.M. (1972) 'Articulation Improvement and Oral Tactile Changes in Children', unpublished Master's thesis, University of West Virginia.

Rutherford, D. and McCall, G. (1967) 'Testing Oral Sensation and Perception in Persons with Dysarthria' in Bosma, J.F. (ed.), *Symposium on Oral Sensation and Perception*, Charles C. Thomas, Springfield, Ill.

Ryan, B.P. (1971) 'Operant Procedures Applied to Stuttering Therapy for Children', *Journal of Speech and Hearing Disorders, 36*, 264-80.

Ryan, B.P. and Van Kirk, B. (1974) 'Re-establishment, Transfer and Maintenance of Fluent Speech in 50 Stutterers Using Delayed Auditory Feedback and Operant Procedures', *Journal of Speech and Hearing Disorders*, *39*, 3-10.

Salvatore, A.P. (1975) 'The Effects of Pause Duration on Sentence Comprehension by Aphasic Individuals', paper presented at the American Speech and Hearing Association Convention, Washington, DC.

Salvatore, A.P. and Brookshire, R.H. (1978) 'The Effects of Pause Placement on Comprehension of Spoken Commands by Aphasic Individuals', paper presented at the American Speech and Hearing Association Convention, San Francisco, California.

Sands, E.S., Freeman, F.J. and Harris, K.S. (1978) 'Progressive Changes in Articulatory Patterns in Verbal Apraxia: a Longitudinal Case Study', *Brain and Language*, *6*, 97-105.

Satz, P. (1976) 'Cerebral Dominance and Reading Disability: an Old Problem Revisited' in Knights, R.M. and Baker, D.J. (eds.), *The Neuropsychology of Learning Disorders*, University Park Press, Baltimore.

Satz, P., Aschenbach, K., Pattishall, E. and Fennell, E. (1965) 'Order of Report, Ear, Asymmetry, and Handedness in Dichotic Listening', *Cortex*, *1*, 377-96.

Schill, M.J. and Schuckers, G.H. (1973) 'Auditory Assembly of Non-prosodic Sentences by Children', *Journal of Communication Disorders*, *6*, 303-14.

Schliesser, H.F. and Coleman, R.O. (1968) 'Effectiveness of Certain Procedures for Alteration of Auditory and Tactile Sensation for Speech', *Perceptual Motor Skills*, *26*, 275-83.

Schuckers, G.H., Shriner, T.H. and Daniloff, R.G. (1973) 'Auditory Reassembly of Segmented Sentences by Children', *Journal of Speech and Hearing Research*, *16*, 116-27.

Schulhoff, C. and Goodglass, H. (1969) 'Dichotic Listening, Side of Brain Injury and Cerebral Dominance', *Neuropsychologia*, *7*, 149-60.

Schwartz, M.F. (1971) 'Acoustic Measures of Nasalization and Nasality' in Grabb, W.C., Rosenstein, S.W. and Bzoch, K.R. (eds.), *Cleft Lip and Palate: Surgical, Dental and Speech Aspects*, Little, Brown and Co., Boston.

Scully, C. (1980) 'Aspects of Nasality in Normal and Abnormal Speech Production', *Proceedings of the 8th Conference of the College of Speech Therapists, Warwick*, 57-68.

Seaver, E.J., Andrews, J.R. and Granata, J.J. (1980) 'A Radiographic Investigation of Velar Positioning in Hearing Impaired Young Adults', *Journal of Communication Disorders*, *13*, 239-47.

Seaver, E.J. and Kuehn, D.P. (1980) 'A Cineradiographic and Electro-myographic Investigation of Velar Positioning in Non-nasal Speech', *Cleft Palate Journal*, *17*, 216-26.

Seebach, M. and Caruso, A. (1979) 'Voice Onset Time During the Fluent Speech of Young Stutterers', paper presented at the American Speech and Hearing Association Convention, Atlanta, Georgia.

Shanks, J. and Ryan, W. (1976) 'A Comparison of Aphasic and Non-brain-injured Adults on a Dichotic CV-syllable Listening Task', *Cortex*, *12*, 100-12.

Shankweiler, D., Harris, K.S. and Taylor, M.L. (1968) 'Electromyographic Studies of Articulation in Aphasia', *Archives of Physical Medicine and Rehabilitation*, *49*, 1-8.

Shankweiler, D. and Studdert-Kennedy, M. (1967) 'Identification of Consonants and Vowels Presented to Left and Right Ears', *Quarterly Journal of Experimental Psychology*, *19*, 59-63.

Sharp, M. and Orchik, D.J. (1978) 'Auditory Function in Sickle Cell Anemia', *Archives of Otolaryngology*, *104*, 332-4.

Shaw, R.E., Folkins, J.W. and Kuehn, D.P. (1980) 'Comparisons of Methods for Measuring Velar Position from Lateral-View Cine-radiography', *Cleft Palate Journal*, *17*, 326-9.

Sheehan, J.G., Aseltine, S. and Edwards, A.E. (1973) 'Aphasic Comprehension of Time Spacing', *Journal of Speech and Hearing Research*, *16*, 650-7.

Shelton, R.L. (1979) 'Oral Sensory Function in Speech Production and Remediation' in Bzoch, K.R. (ed.), *Communicative Disorders Related to Cleft Lip and Palate* (2nd edn), Little Brown and Company, Boston, Mass.

Shelton, R.L., Arndt, W.B. and Hetherington, J.J. (1967) 'Testing Oral Stereognosis' in Bosma, J.F. (ed.), *Symposium on Oral Sensation and Perception*, Charles C. Thomas, Springfield, Ill.

Shelton, R.L., Beaumont, K.B., Trier, W.C. and Furr, M.L. (1978) 'Videopanandoscopic Feedback in Training Velopharyngeal Closure', *Cleft Palate Journal*, *15*, 6-12.

Shelton, R.L., Furr, M.L., Johnson, A. and Arndt, W.B. (1975) 'Cephalometric and Intra-oral Variables as they Relate to Articulation Improvement with Training', *American Journal of Orthodontics*, *67*, 423-31.

Shelton, R.L., Knox, A.W., Elbert, M. and Johnson, T.S. (1970) 'Palate Awareness and Non Speech Voluntary Palate Movement' in Bosma, J.F. (ed.), *Second Symposium on Oral Sensation and Perception*, Charles C. Thomas, Springfield, Ill.

Shelton, R.L. and Trier, W.C. (1976) 'Issues Involved in the Evaluation of Velopharyngeal Closure', *Cleft Palate Journal*, *13*, 127-37.

Shelton, R.L., Willis, V., Johnson, A.F. and Arndt, W.B. (1973) 'Oral Form Recognition Training and Articulation Change', *Perceptual Motor Skills*, *26*, 523-31.

Shipp, T. and McGlone, R.E. (1971) 'Laryngeal Dynamics Associated with Voice Frequency Changes', *Journal of Speech and Hearing Research*, *14*, 761-8.

Shoup, J.E. and Pfeifer, L.L. (1976) 'Acoustic Characteristics of Speech Sounds' in Lass, N.J. (ed.), *Contemporary Issues in Experimental Phonetics*, Academic Press, New York.

Shprintzen, R.J., Croft, C.B., Berkman, M.D. and Rakoff, S.J. (1980) 'Velopharyngeal Insufficiency in the Facio-Auriculo-Vertebral Malformation Complex', *Cleft Palate Journal*, *17*, 132-7.

Shprintzen, R.J., McCall, G.N. and Skolnick, M.L. (1975) 'A New Therapeutic Technique for the Treatment of Velopharyngeal Incompetence', *Journal of Speech and Hearing Disorders*, *40*, 69-83.

Shriner, T.H. and Daniloff, R.G. (1970) 'Reassembly of Segmented CVC Syllables by Children', *Journal of Speech and Hearing Research*, *13*, 537-47.

Siegel, G.M. , Fehst, C.A., Garber, S.R. and Pick, H.L. (1980) 'Delayed Auditory Feedback with Children', *Journal of Speech and Hearing Research*, *23*, 802-13.

Silverman, S. and Hirsh, I. (1955) 'Problems Related to the Use of Speech in Clinical Audiometry', *Annals of Otology, Rhinology and Laryngology*, *64*, 1234-44.

Simpson, R.K. and Colton, J. (1980) 'A Cephalometric Study of Velar Stretch in Adolescent Subjects', *Cleft Palate Journal*, *17*, 40-7.

Singh, S. and Schlanger, B. (1969) 'Effects of Delayed Sidetone on the Speech of Aphasic, Dysarthric, and Mentally Retarded Subjects', *Language and Speech*, *12*, 167-74.

Smith, J.L. (1977) *Mechanisms of Neuromuscular Control*, UCLA Printing and Production, Los Angeles, Ca.

Smith, J.L., Roberts, E.M. and Atkins, E. (1972) 'Fusimotor Neuron Block and Voluntary Arm Movement in Man', *American Journal of Physical Medicine*, *5*, 225-39.

Smith, R.M. (1964) 'Stereognosis Perception Within the Mouths of Children with Speech Problems', unpublished Master of Education research paper, Pennsylvania State University.

Snidecor, J.C. and Curry, E.T. (1959) 'Temporal and Pitch Aspects of Superior Oesophageal Speech', *Annals of Otolaryngology*, *68*, 623-36.

Snidecor, J.C. and Isshiki, N. (1965) 'Air Volume and Airflow Relationships of Six Male Oesophageal Speakers', *Journal of Speech and Hearing Disorders*, *30*, 205-16.

Snow, J., Rintelmann, W.F., Miller, J. and Konkle, D.F. (1977) 'Central Auditory Imperception', *Laryngoscope*, *87*, 1450-71.

Soderberg, G. (1969) 'Delayed Auditory Feedback and the Speech of Stutterers', *Journal of Speech and Hearing Disorders*, *33*, 20-9.

Sommers, R.K., Brady, W.A. and Moore, W.H. Jr. (1975) 'Dichotic Ear Preferences of Stuttering Children and Adults', *Perceptual and Motor Skills*, *41*, 931-8.

Sommers, R.K., Cox, S. and West, C. (1972) 'Articulatory Effectiveness, Stimulability and Children's Performances on Perceptual and Memory Tasks', *Journal of Speech and Hearing Research*, *15*, 579-89.

Sommers, R.K., Moore, W.H. Jnr., Brady, W.A. and Jackson, P. (1972) 'Performance of Articulatory Defective, Minimal Brain Dysfunctioning, and Normal Children on Dichotic Ear Preference, Laterality, and Fine-motor Tasks', *Journal of Special Education*, *10*, 5-14.

Sommers, R.K. and Starkey, K.L. (1977) 'Dichotic Verbal Processing in Down's Syndrome Children Having Qualitatively Different Speech and Language Skills', *American Journal of Mental Deficiency*, *82*, 44-53.

Sommers, R.K. and Taylor, M.L. (1972) 'Cerebral Speech Dominance in Language-Disordered and Normal Children', *Cortex*, *8*, 224-32.

Sparks, R. and Geschwind, N. (1968) 'Dichotic Listening in Man after Section of Neocortical Commissures', *Cortex*, *4*, 3-16.

Sparks, R., Goodglass, H. and Nickel, B. (1970) 'Ipsilateral Versus Contralateral Extinction in Dichotic Listening Resulting from Hemispheric Lesions', *Cortex*, *6*, 249-60.

Speaks, C., Carney, E., Niccum, N. and Johnson, C. (1981) 'Stimulus Dominance in Dichotic Listening', *Journal of Speech and Hearing Research*, *24*, 430-7.

Speaks, C. and Jerger, J. (1965) 'Method for Measurement of Speech Identification', *Journal of Speech and Hearing Research*, *8*, 185-94.

Spoor, A. and Van Dishoeck, H.A. (1960) 'Electromyography of the Human Vocal Cords and the Theory of Husson', *Practical Otorinolaryngology*, *20*, 353-60.

Stanton, J.B. (1958) 'The Effects of DAF on the Speech of Aphasic Patients', *Scottish Medical Journal*, *3*, 378-84.

Starkey, K. (1974) 'The Dichotic Testing of Young Children: a New Test for the Speech and Hearing Impaired', unpublished Masters thesis, Kent State University, Ohio.

Steer, M. (1937) 'Symptomatology of Young Stutterers', *Journal of Speech Disorders*, 2, 3-13.

Stetson, R.H. (1937) 'Oesophageal Speech for any Laryngectomised Patient', *Archives of Otolaryngology*, 26, 132-42.

Stevens, K.N. and House, A.S. (1955) 'Development of a Quantitative Description of Vowel Articulation', *Journal of the Acoustical Society of America*, 27, 484-93.

Stevens, K.N. and House, A.S. (1961) 'An Acoustical Theory of Vowel Production and Some of its Implications', *Journal of Speech and Hearing Research*, 4, 303-20.

Sticht, T.G. (1969) 'Learning by Listening in Relation to Aptitude, Reading and Rate-controlled Speech', *Hum RRO Technical Report 69-23*, Department of the Army.

Sticht, T.G. and Gray, B.B. (1969) 'The Intelligibility of Time-compressed Words as a Function of Age and Hearing Loss', *Journal of Speech and Hearing Research*, 12, 443-8.

Stoyva, J. (1977) 'Self-regulation and the Stress-related Disorders: a Perspective on Biofeedback' in Kamiya, J. *Biofeedback and Self-Control*, Aldine, Chicago.

Strenger, F. (1968) 'Radiographic, Palatographic, and Labiographic Methods in Phonetics' in Malmberg, B. (ed.), *Manual of Phonetics*, North Holland, Amsterdam.

Strother, C. (1935) 'A Study of the Extent of Dyssynergia Occurring During the Stuttering Spasm', unpublished PhD thesis, State University of Iowa.

Stuart, D.G., Mosher, C.G., Gerlack, R.L. and Reinking, R.M. (1972) 'Mechanical Arrangement and Transducing Properties of Golgi Tendon Organs', *Experimental Brain Research*, 14, 274-92.

Studdert-Kennedy, M. and Shankweiler, D. (1970) 'Hemispheric Specialization for Speech Perception', *Journal of the Acoustical Society of America*, 48, 579-94.

Subtelny, J.D., Oya, N. and Subtelny, J.D. (1972) 'Cineradiographic Study of Sibilants', *Folia Phoniatrica*, 24, 30-50.

Sussman, H.M. (1972) 'What the Tongue Tells the Brain', *Psychological Bulletin*, 77, 262-72.

Sussman, H.M. and MacNeilage, P.F. (1975) 'Hemispheric Specialization for Speech Production and Perception in Stutterers', *Neuropsychologia*, 13, 19-27.

Tallal, P. and Newcombe, F. (1978) 'Impairment of Auditory Perception and Language Comprehension in Dysphasia', *Brain and Language*, 5, 13-24.

Teixeira, L.A., Defran, R.H. and Nichols, A.C. (1974) 'Oral Stereognostic Differences Between Apraxics, Dysarthrics, Aphasics and Normals', *Journal of Communication Disorders*, 7, 213-25.

Telage, K.M. and Fucci, D.J. (1973) 'Vibrotactile Stimulation: a Future Clinical Tool for Speech Pathologists', *Journal of Speech and Hearing Disorders*, 38, 442-7.

Telage, K.M. and Fucci, D.J. (1974) 'Concerning Intrasubject Measurements of Successive Lingual Vibrotactile Responses', *Perceptual Motor Skills*, 39, 1047-52.

Thompson, N.W. (1973) 'Comprehension of Rate-controlled Speech of Varying Linguistic Complexity by Normal Children', paper presented at the American Speech and Hearing Association Convention, Detroit, Michigan.

Tiffany, W., Hanley, C. and Sutherland, L. (1954) 'A Simple Mechanical Adaptor for Variable Sidetone Delay', *Journal of Speech and Hearing Disorders*, 19, 504-6.

Tillman, T. and Carhart, R. (1966) 'An Expanded Test for Speech Discrimination using CNC Monosyllable Words (N.U. Auditory Test No. 6)', *Technical Report No. SAM-RT-66-55*, U.S.A. Air Force School of Aerospace Medicine, Brooks Air Force Base, Texas.

Timmons, B. and Boudreau, J. (1972) 'Auditory Feedback as a Major Factor in Stuttering', *Journal of Speech and Hearing Disorders, 37*, 476-84.

Tingley, B.M., and Allen, G.D. (1975) 'Development of Speech Timing Control in Children', *Child Development*, 46, 186-94.

Torrans, A. and Beasley, D.S. (1975) 'Oral Stereognosis: Effect of Varying Form Set, Answer Type and Retention Time', *Journal of Psycholinguistic Research*, 2, 159-67.

Travis, L.E. (1931) *Speech Pathology*, Appleton-Century, New York.

Travis, L.E. (1934) 'Disassociation of the Homologous Muscle Function in Stutterers', *Archives of Neurology and Psychiatry, 31*, 127-33.

Tzavaras, A., Kaprinis, G. and Gatzoyas, A. (1981) 'Literacy and Hemispheric Specialization for Language: Digit Dichotic Listening in Illiterates', *Neuropsychologia*, 19, 565-70.

Umeda, N. (1975) 'Vowel Duration in American English', *Journal of the Acoustical Society of America*, 58, 434-45.

Van den Berg, J. (1955) 'On the Role of the Laryngeal Ventricle in

Voice Production', *Folia Phoniatrica*, 7, 57-69.

Van den Berg, J., Moolenar-Bijl, A.J. and Damste, P.H. (1958) 'Oesophageal Speech', *Folia Phoniatrica*, 10, 65-84.

Van der Plaats, G.J. (1969) *Medical X-Ray Technique*, Centrex Publishing Company, Eindhoven.

Van Gelder, L. (1974) 'Psychosomatic Aspects of Endocrine Disorders of the Voice', *Journal of Communication Disorders*, 7, 257-62.

Van Ort, D., Beasley, D.S. and Riensche, L.L. (1979) 'Intelligibility of Time-altered Sentential Messages as a Function of Contralateral Masking' in Hollien, H. and Hollien, P. (eds.), *Current Issues in the Phonetic Sciences*, Part IV, vol. 9.

Van Riper, C. (1954) *Speech Correction: Principles and Methods*, Prentice-Hall, Englewood Cliffs, NJ.

Van Riper, C. (1970) 'The Use of DAF in Stuttering Therapy', *British Journal of Disorders of Communication*, 5, 40-5.

Van Riper, C. (1971) *The Nature of Stuttering*, Prentice-Hall, Englewood Cliffs, NJ.

Van Riper, C. (1973) *The Treatment of Stuttering*, Prentice-Hall, Englewood Cliffs, NJ.

Van Riper, C. and Irwin, J.V. (1958) *Voice and Articulation*, Prentice-Hall, Englewood Cliffs, NJ.

Venkatagiri, H.S. (1980) 'The Relevance of DAF-induced Speech Disruption to the Understanding of Stuttering', *Journal of Fluency Disorders*, 5, 87-98.

Vincent, T. and Bradshaw, J. (1975) 'A Simple Device for the Preparation of Exactly Aligned Dichotic Tapes', *Behavior Research Methods and Instrumentation*, 7, 534-8.

Vrtunski, P.B., Mack, J.L., Boller, F. and Kim, Y.C. (1976) 'Response to Delayed Auditory Feedback in Patients with Hemispheric Lesions', *Cortex*, 12, 395-404.

Ward, P.H., Hanafee, W., Shallit, J., Mancuso, A. and Berci, G. (1979) 'Evaluation of Computerized Tomography, Cinelaryngoscopy, and Laryngography in Determining the Extent of Laryngeal Disease', *Annals of Otology, Rhinology and Laryngology*, 88, 454-62.

Warren, D.W. and Ryon, W.E. (1967) 'Oral Port Constriction, Nasal Resistance and Respiratory Aspects of Cleft-Palate Speech; an Analogue Study', *Cleft Palate Journal*, 4, 38-46.

Webster, R.L. and Lubker, B.B. (1968) 'Interrelationships Among Fluency Producing Variables in Stuttered Speech', *Journal of Speech and Hearing Research*, 11, 754-66.

Wechsler, E. (1976a) 'Laryngographic Study of Voice Disorders',

Speech and Hearing: Work in Progress, UCL, London.

Wechsler, E. (1976b) 'The Use of the Laryngograph in the Study of some Patients with Voice Disorders', unpublished MSc thesis, University of London.

Wechsler, E. (1977) 'Laryngographic Study of Voice Disorders', *British Journal of Disorders of Communication*, *12*, 9-22.

Weddell, G., Feinstein, B. and Pattle, R.E. (1944) 'The Electrical Activity of Voluntary Muscle in Man Under Normal and Pathological Conditions', *Brain*, *67*, 178.

Weidner, W.E. and Lasky, E.Z. (1976) 'The Interaction of Rate and Complexity of Stimulus on the Performance of Adult Aphasic Subjects', *Brain and Language*, *3*, 34-40.

Weinberg, B. (1981) 'Speech Alternatives Following Total Laryngectomy' in Darby, J.K. (ed.), *Speech Evaluation in Medicine*, Grune and Stratton, New York.

Weinberg, B., Liss, G.M. and Hillis, J.A. (1970) 'Comparative Study of Visual Manual and Oral Form Identification Skills in Speech Impaired and Normal Speaking Children' in Bosma, J.F. (ed.), *Second Symposium on Oral Sensation and Perception*, Charles C. Thomas, Springfield, Ill.

Weinberg, B., Lyons, M.J. and Liss, G.M. (1970) 'Studies of Oral Manual and Visual Form Identification Skills in Children and Adults' in Bosma, J.F. (ed.), *Second Symposium on Oral Sensation and Perception*, Charles C. Thomas, Springfield, Ill.

Weiss, C. and Blackley, F. (1981) 'Feasibility of Using Computerized Tomography in Diagnosing Nasopharyngeal Closure', *Journal of Communication Disorders*, *14*, 43-50.

Weiss, M.J. and House, A.S. (1973) 'Perception of Dichotically Presented Vowels', *Journal of the Acoustical Society of America*, *38*, 583-9.

Wernicke, C. (1908) 'The Symptom-complex of Aphasia' in Church, A. (ed.), *Diseases of the Nervous System*, Appleton, London.

Wetzel, M.C. and Stuart, D.G. (1976) 'Ensemble Characteristics of Cat Locomotion and its Neural Control', *Progress in Neurobiology*, *7*, 1-98.

Wexler, B., Halwes, T. and Heninger, G. (1981) 'Use of Statistical Significance Criterion in Drawing Inferences About Hemispheric Dominance for Language Function from Dichotic Listening Data', *Brain and Language*, *13*, 13-18.

Whetnall, E. and Fry, D.B. (1964) *The Deaf Child*, William Heinemann Medical Books, London.

Wilhelm, C.L. (1971) 'The Effects of Oral Form Recognition Training on Articulation in Children', unpublished Doctoral dissertation, University of Kansas.

Willeford, J. (1976) 'Central Auditory Function' in Donnelly, K. (ed.), *Communicative Disorders: Learning Disabilities*, Little, Brown and Co, New York.

Williams, D.E. (1955) 'Masseter Muscle Action Potentials in Stuttered and Non-stuttered Speech', *Journal of Speech and Hearing Disorders, 20*, 242-61.

Williams, W.N. (1971) 'Applications of Radiological Measures' in Grabb, W.C., Rosenstein, S.W. and Bzoch, K.R. (eds.), *Cleft Lip and Palate*, Little, Brown and Co, Boston.

Williams, W.N. and Eisenbach, C.R. (1981) 'Assessing VP Function: the Lateral Still Technique vs Cinefluorography', *Cleft Palate Journal, 18*, 45-50.

Williams, W.N. and LaPointe, L.L. (1971) 'Intra-oral Recognition of Geometric Forms by Normal Subjects', *Perceptual Motor Skills, 32*, 419-26.

Wilsher, C.R. (1981) 'Right Hemisphere Dominant or Left Hemisphere Dysfunction', *Dyslexia Review, 4*, 5-7.

Wirz, S. and Anthony, J. (1979) 'The Use of the Voiscope in Improving the Speech of Profoundly Deaf Children', *British Journal of Disorders of Communication, 14*, 137-52.

Wirz, S.L., Subtelny, J.D. and Whitehead, R.L. (1981) 'Perceptual and Spectrographic Study of Tense Voice in Normal Hearing and Deaf Subjects', *Folia Phoniatrica, 33*, 23-36.

Witelson, S. (1976) 'Sex and the Single Hemisphere: Specialization of the Right Hemisphere for Spatial Processing', *Science, 193*, 426-7.

Witelson, S. (1977) 'Developmental Dyslexia: Two Right Hemispheres and None Left', *Science, 195*, 309-11.

Wolfe, V.I. and Bacon, M. (1976) 'Spectrographic Comparison of Two Types of Spastic Dysphonia', *Journal of Speech and Hearing Disorders, 41*, 325-33.

Woodford, L.D. (1964) 'Oral Stereognosis', unpublished Master's thesis in Orthodontics, University of Illinois.

Yairi, E. and Cavaness, D. (1975) 'Successive Versus Simultaneous Presentation of Forms in Oral Stereognostic Testing', *Perceptual Motor Skills, 41*, 233-4.

Yanagihara, N. (1967a) 'Hoarseness: Investigation of the Physiological Mechanisms', *Annals of Otology, Rhinology and Laryngology, 76*, 427-88.

Yanagihara, N. (1967b) 'Significance of Harmonic Changes and Noise Components in Hoarseness', *Journal of Speech and Hearing Research*, *10*, 531-41.

Yanagihara, N. and von Leden, H. (1967) 'Respiration and Phonation', *Folia Phoniatrica*, *19*, 153-66.

Yates, A, (1963) 'Delayed Auditory Feedback', *Psychological Bulletin*, *60*, 213-32.

Yeni-Komshian, G.H. and Gordon, J.F. (1974) 'The Effects of Memory Load on the Right Ear Advantage in Dichotic Listening', *Brain and Language*, *1*, 375-81.

Zawadski, P.A. and Kuehn, D.P. (1980) 'A Cineradiographic Study of Static and Dynamic Aspects of American English /r/', *Phonetica*, *37*, 253-66.

Zimmerman, G. (1980a) 'Articulatory Dynamics of Fluent Utterances of Stutterers and Nonstutterers', *Journal of Speech and Hearing Research*, *23*, 95-107.

Zimmerman, G. (1980b) 'Articulatory Behaviors Associated with Stuttering: a Cinefluorographic Analysis', *Journal of Speech and Hearing Research*, *23*, 108-21.

Zimmerman, G. (1980c) 'Stuttering: a Disorder of Movement', *Journal of Speech and Hearing Research*, *23*, 122-36.

Zimmerman, G., Kelso, J.A.S. and Lander, L. (1980) 'Articulatory Behavior Pre and Post Full-mouth Tooth Extraction and Alveoplasty: a Cinefluorographic Study', *Journal of Speech and Hearing Research*, *23*, 630-45.

Zimmerman, S.A. and Sapon, S.M. (1958) 'Note on Vowel Duration Seen Cross-linguistically', *Journal of the Acoustical Society of America*, *30*, 152-3.

Zwitman, D.H., Gyepes, M.T. and Ward, P.H. (1976) 'Assessment of Velar and Lateral Wall Movement by Oral Telescope and Radiographic Investigation in Patients with Velopharyngeal Inadequacy and in Normal Subjects', *Journal of Speech and Hearing Disorders*, *41*, 381-9.

INDEX